TNM Atlas

Illustrated Guide to the TNM Classification
of Malignant Tumours

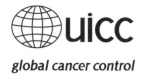

global cancer control

TNM Atlas

Illustrated Guide to the TNM Classification of Malignant Tumours

5th Edition

Editors
Ch. Wittekind, F. L. Greene, R. V. P. Hutter,
M. Klimpfinger and L. H. Sobin

With 505 Illustrations

WILEY-LISS

A JOHN WILEY & SONS, INC., PUBLICATION

Prof. Dr. Ch. Wittekind
Direktor des Institutes für Pathologie
Universität Leipzig,
Liebigstr. 26
D-04103 Leipzig

Dr. F. L. Greene
Carolinas Medical Center
Department of Surgery
1000 Blythe Boulevard
Charlotte, NC 28203, USA

Dr. R. V. P. Hutter
30 Surrey Lane
Livingston, NJ 07039, USA

Dr. L. H. Sobin
Department of Gastrointestinal and
Hepatic Pathology
Armed Forces Institute of Pathology,
Washington, DC 20306, USA

Prof. Dr. M. Klimpfinger
Vorstand des Pathologischen und
bakteriologischen Institutes
Kaiser-Franz-Josef-Spital
Kundratstrasse 3
A-110 Vienna

Published by John Wiley & Sons, Inc., Hoboken, New Jersey.
Published simultaneously in Canada.

For general information on our other products and services or for technical support, please contact our Customer Care Department within the United States at (800) 762-2974, outside the United States at (317) 572-3993 or fax (317) 572-4002.

Wiley also publishes its books in a variety of electronic formats. Some content that appears in print may not be available in electronic formats. For more information about Wiley products, visit our web site at www.wiley.com.

Library of Congress Cataloging-in-Publication Data is available.

ISBN-13 978-0-471-74301-9
ISBN-10 0-471-74301-1

Printed in the United States of America.

10 9 8 7 6 5 4 3 2 1

Contents

Preface to the Fifth Edition

This new fifth edition of the TNM Atlas reflects the changes in the TNM System introduced by the recently published 6th edition of the TNM Classification of Malignant Tumours [1]. The most important additions and modifications are:

- A revised classification of head and neck tumours reflecting the introduction of T4a/pT4a and T4b/pT4b categories, which allow a ramification in locally operable and nonoperable tumours
- A new classification of tumours of the nasal cavity
- Changes in the classification of thyroid tumours
- New subcategories in the classification of gastric tumours
- Changes in the classifications of tumours of the liver, gallbladder, extrahepatic bile ducts, liver, and pancreas
- A new classification of malignant mesothelioma of pleura
- Changes in the classification of bone tumours
- Substantial changes in the classification of malignant melanoma of the skin
- Changes in the classification of regional lymph nodes of the breast
- Modifications in the definition of risk factors of gestational trophoblastic tumours according to the proposals of FIGO
- New subcategories in the classification of tumours of the prostate
- Changes in the classifications of ophthalmic tumours

Additionally, a proposal for the classification of sentinel lymph nodes was introduced as well as a classification of isolated tumour cells (ITC) in regional lymph nodes and bone marrow.

The editorial board has changed: Dr. Hermanek, the editor-in-chief of the former edition and one of the "fathers" of the TNM Atlas, has retired, as has Dr. Wagner; Dr. Klimpfinger has joined the board. The editors wish to express many thanks to Paul Hermanek for his great contributions to the development and promotion of the TNM Atlas and to Dr. Wagner for his valuable work.

The editorial board has tried to follow the innovative concept developed by Bernd Spiessl to provide a graphic aid for the practical application of the TNM classification system. The TNM classification, as presented and illustrated in this edition, corresponds exactly to the 6th edition of the UICC TNM Classification of Malignant Tumours [1] and the 6th edition of the AJCC Cancer Staging Manual [2]. Recent modifications by FIGO [3] are also included in order to keep the FIGO and TNM classifications identical.

Substantial changes between the revised fourth edition (1998) and the present edition of the TNM Atlas are indicated by a line at the left-hand side of the page.

The editors hope that the TNM Atlas will continue to facilitate the daily practice of oncologists and to enhance the use of TNM in planning treatment, estimating prognosis and evaluating treatment results.

Ch. Wittekind, Leipzig
F. L. Greene, Charlotte, NC
R. V. P. Hutter, Livingston, NJ
L. H. Sobin, Washington, DC
M. Klimpfinger, Vienna

February 2005

References

1. UICC: TNM Classification of Malignant Tumours. 6th edition (2002). Sobin LH, Wittekind Ch (eds). Wiley, New York
2. Greene FL, Balch CM, Fleming ID, Fritz A, Haller DG, Morrow M, Page DL (eds) (2002) AJCC Cancer Staging Manual, 6th ed. Springer, New York
3. Creasman WT, Odicino F, Maisoneuve P, Beller U, Benedet JL, Heintz APM, Ngan HYS, Sideri M, Pecorelli S (2001) FIGO Annual report on the results and treatment in gynaecological cancer, vol 24. Carcinoma of the corpus uteri. J Epidemiol Biostat 6:45–86

Foreword to the First Edition

Confronted with a myriad of T's, N's and M's in the UICC TNM booklet, classifying a malignancy may seem to many cancer clinicians a tedious, dull and pedantic task. But with a look at the TNM Atlas all of a sudden lifeless categories become vivid images, challenging the clinicians's know-how and investigational skills.

Brigit van der Werf-Messing, M. D.
Professor of Radiology
Chairman of the International TNM Committee of the UICC

Rotterdam, July 1982

Acknowledgements

The editors wish to express their thanks to Prof. Dr. Dr. h. c. Paul Hermanek, Erlangen, for his invaluable help in the preparation of the manuscript and illustrations.

They are equally grateful to Mr. P. Lübke who took great care in drawing the anatomical illustrations.

Funding of the TNM Project by the Centers for Disease Control and Prevention (USA) through grant HR3/CCH417470 is gratefully acknowledged. The content of the publication is solely the responsibility of the authors and does not necessarily represent the official views of the CDC.

Contributors to the Fifth Edition

Bootz, F., Leipzig, FRG   Head and Neck Surgery
Hermanek, P., Erlangen, FRG   Pathology
Sobin, L. H., Washington/DC, USA   Pathology
Spraul, Ch., Ulm, FRG   Ophthalmology
Weber, Anette, Leipzig, FRG   Head and Neck Surgery
Wittekind, Ch., Leipzig, FRG   Pathology

Contributors to the Fourth Edition

Bootz F., Leipzig, FRG — Head and neck surgery
Hermanek P., Erlangen, FRG — Pathology
Howaldt H. J., Gießen, FRG — Head and neck surgery
Hutter R. V. P., Livingston, NJ, USA — Pathology
Paterok E., Erlangen, FRG — Gynaecology
Sobin L. H., Washington, DC, USA — Pathology
Wagner G., Heidelberg, FRG — Documentation and Epidemiology

Wittekind Ch., Leipzig, FRG — Pathology

Contributors to the Third Edition

Baker, H. W., Portland, OR, USA — Head and neck surgery
Beahrs, O. H., Rochester, MN, USA — General surgery
Drepper, H., Münster-Handorf, FRG — Maxillofacial surgery
Gemsenjäger, E., Basel, Switzerland — General surgery
Genz, T., Berlin FRG — Gynaecology
Glanz, H., Marburg, FRG — Otorhinolaryngology
Hasse, J., Freiburg, FRG — Thoracic surgery
Hermanek, P., Erlangen, FRG — Pathology
Hutter, R. V. P., Livingston, NJ, USA — Pathology
Kindermann, G., München, FRG — Gynaecology
Kleinsasser, O., Marburg, FRG — Otorhinolaryngology
Lang, G., Erlangen, FRG — Ophthalmology
Naumann, G. O. H., Erlangen, FRG — Ophthalmology
Remagen, W., Basel, Switzerland — Pathology
Scheibe, O., Stuttgart, FRG — General surgery
Schmitt, H. P., Heidelberg, FRG — Neuropathology
Sobin, L. H., Washington, DC, USA — Pathology
Spiessl, B., Basel, Switzerland — Maxillofacial surgery
Wagner, G., Heidelberg, FRG — Documentation and Epidemiology

Contributors to the Second Edition

Adolphs, H. D., Höxter, FRG — Urology

Amberger, H., Heidelberg, FRG — General surgery

Baumann, R. P., Neuchâtel, Switzerland — Pathology

Berger, H., Göttingen, FRG — Dermatology

Bokelmann, D., Essen, FRG — General surgery

Brandeis, W. F., Heidelberg, FRG — Paediatric oncology

Dold, U., Gauting, FRG — Internal medicine

Drepper, H., Münster-Handorf, FRG — Maxillofacial surgery

Drings, P., Heidelberg, FRG — Internal medicine

Gemsenjäger, E., Basel, Switzerland — General surgery

Hasse, J., Basel, Switzerland — Thoracic surgery

Heitz, Ph., Basel, Switzerland — Pathology

Hermanek, P., Erlangen, FRG — Pathology

Karrer, K., Wien, Austria — Oncological epidemiology

Kuehnl-Petzold, C. Freiburg i.Br., FRG — Dermatology

Liebenstein, J., Mannheim, FRG — Gynaecology

Molitor, D., Bonn, FRG — Urology

Nidecker, A., Basel, Switzerland — Radiology

Rohde, H., Köln, FRG — General surgery

Scheibe, O., Stuttgart, FRG — General surgery

Schmitt, A., Mannheim, FRG — Gynaecology

Spiessl, B., Basel, Switzerland — Maxillofacial surgery

Thomas, C., Marburg, FRG — Pathology

Vogt-Moykopf, I., Heidelberg, FRG — Thoracic surgery

Wagner, G., Heidelberg, FRG — Documentation and Epidemiology

Preliminary Note[1]

The TNM System for describing the anatomical extent of disease is based an assessment of three components:

T – The extent of the primary tumour
N – The absence or presence and extent of regional lymph node metastasis
M – The absence or presence of distant metastasis

The addition of numbers to these three components indicates the extent of the malignant disease, thus:

T0, T1, T2, T3, T4 N0, N 1, N2, N3 M0, M1

In effect, the System is a "shorthand notation" for describing the extent of a particular malignant tumour.

Each site is described under the following headings:

1. *Anatomy.*
   Drawings of the anatomical sites and subsites are presented with the appropriate ICD-O topography numbers.[1]
2. *Regional Lymph Nodes.*
   The regional lymph nodes are listed and shown in drawings.
3. *T/pT Clinical and Pathological Classification of the Primary Tumour.*
   The definitions for T and pT categories are presented. In the sixth edition (2002) of the TNM Classification the clinical and pathological classification (T and pT) generally coincide, therefore the same illustrations are valid for the T and pT classification. The only exceptions to this are malignant melanoma of uvea and conjunctiva, as well as retinoblastoma.
4. *N/pN Clinical and Pathological Classification of Regional Lymph Nodes.*
   The N and pN categories are presented in a fashion similar to the T and pT categories. Differences between N and pN definitions in the sixth edition arise only in the case of carcinoma of the breast and germ cell tumours of the testis.
5. *M/pM Clinical and Pathological Classification of Distant Metastasis.*
   M localization is given only in selected cases because of its many possible variables.

[1] ICD-O International Classification of Diseases for Oncology, 3rd edn(2000), WHO, Geneva

TNM Atlas: Illustrated Guide to the TNM Classification of Malignant Tumours, Fifth Edition,
edited by Christian Wittekind, Frederick L. Greene, Robert Hutter, Martin Klimpfinger, and Leslie H. Sobin
Copyright © 2005 UICC

C Factor

The C factor, or certainty factor, reflects the validity of classification according to the diagnostic methods employed. Its use is optional.

The C-factor definitions are:

C1   Evidence from standard diagnostic means (e.g., inspection, palpation, and standard radiography, intraluminal endoscopy for tumours of certain regions)

C2   Evidence obtained by special diagnostic means, e.g., radiographic imaging in special projections, tomography, computed tomography (CT), ultrasonography, lymphography, angiography; scintigraphy; magnetic resonance imaging (MRI); endoscopy, biopsy, and cytology

C3   Evidence from surgical exploration, including biopsy and cytology

C4   Evidence of the extent of disease following definitive surgery and pathological examination of the resected specimen

C5   Evidence from autopsy

Example

Degrees of C may be applied to the T, N, and M categories. A case might be described as T3C2, N2C1, M0C2.

The TNM clinical classification is therefore equivalent to C1, C2, and C3 in varying degrees of certainty, while the pTNM pathological classification generally is equivalent to C4.

Residual Tumour (R) Classification

The absence or presence of residual tumour after treatment is described by the symbol R. TNM and pTNM describe the anatomical extent of cancer in general without considering treatment. They can be supplemented by the R classification, which deals with tumour status after treatment. The R classification reflects the effects of therapy, influences further therapeutic procedures and is a strong predictor of prognosis.

In the R classification, not only local-regional residual tumour is to be taken into consideration, but also distant residual tumour in the form of remaining distant metastases.

The definitions of the R categories are:

RX   Presence of residual tumour cannot be assessed
R0   No residual tumour (Fig. 1)
R1   Microscopic residual tumour (Fig. 2)
R2   Macroscopic residual tumour (Fig. 3)

TNM Atlas: Illustrated Guide to the TNM Classification of Malignant Tumours, Fifth Edition,
edited by Christian Wittekind, Frederick L. Greene, Robert Hutter, Martin Klimpfinger, and Leslie H. Sobin
Copyright © 2005 UICC

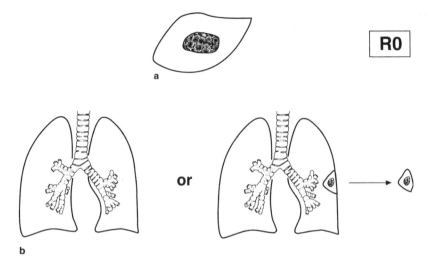

R0

Fig. 1a-c. R0: **a** Primary tumour excised, resection margins without tumour. **b** No distant metastasis or distant metastasis completely removed

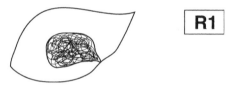

R1

Fig. 2. R1. Excision of the primary tumour grossly complete, but histological examination demonstrates tumour at resection margins

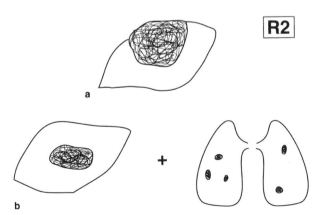

R2

Fig. 3a, b. R2. **a** Grossly incomplete excision of the primary tumour or **b** complete excision of the primary tumour with remaining distant metastases

Head and Neck Tumours

Introductory Notes

The following sites are included:

- Lip, oral cavity
- Pharynx: Oropharynx, nasopharynx, hypopharynx
- Larynx: Supraglottis, glottis, subglottis
- Maxillary sinus
- Nasal cavity, ethmoid sinus
- Salivary gland(s)
- Thyroid gland

Carcinomas arising in minor salivary glands of the upper aerodigestive tract are classified according to the rules for tumours of their anatomic site of origin, e.g., oral cavity.

Substantial changes in the 5th edition compared to the 4th edition are marked by a bar at the left-hand side of the page. The same is true for new classifications of previously unclassified tumours.

TNM Atlas: Illustrated Guide to the TNM Classification of Malignant Tumours, Fifth Edition,
edited by Christian Wittekind, Frederick L. Greene, Robert Hutter, Martin Klimpfinger, and Leslie H. Sobin
Copyright © 2005 UICC

Regional Lymph Nodes (Fig. 4)

The definitions of the N categories for all head and neck sites except nasopharynx and thyroid are the same. These include:

(1) submental nodes
(2) submandibular nodes
(3) cranial jugular (deep cervical) nodes
(4) medial jugular (deep cervical) nodes
(5) caudal jugular (deep cervical) nodes
(6) dorsal cervical (superficial cervical) nodes along the accessory nerve
(7) supraclavicular nodes
(8) prelaryngeal, pretracheal, and paratracheal nodes
(9) retropharyngeal nodes
(10) parotid nodes
(11) buccal nodes
(12) retroauricular and occipital nodes

Note
* The pretracheal lymph nodes are sometimes addressed as "Delphian nodes".

N/pN Classification—Regional Lymph Nodes

The definitions of the N and pN categories for all head and neck sites except nasopharynx and thyroid gland are:

NX/pNX Regional lymph nodes cannot be assessed
N0/pN0 No regional lymph node metastasis

pN0   Histological examination of a selective neck dissection specimen will ordi-
           narily include 6 or more lymph nodes. Histological examination of a radical
           or modified radical neck dissection specimen will ordinarily include 10
           or more lymph nodes. If the lymph nodes are negative, but the number
           ordinarily examined is not met, classify as pN0.
           When size is a criterion for pN classification, measurement is made of the
           metastasis, not of the entire lymph node.

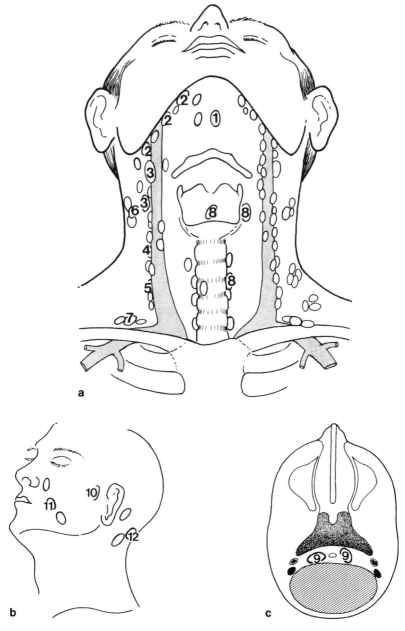

Fig. 4a-c

N1/pN1   Metastasis in a single ipsilateral lymph node, 3 cm or less in greatest
          dimension (Fig. 5)

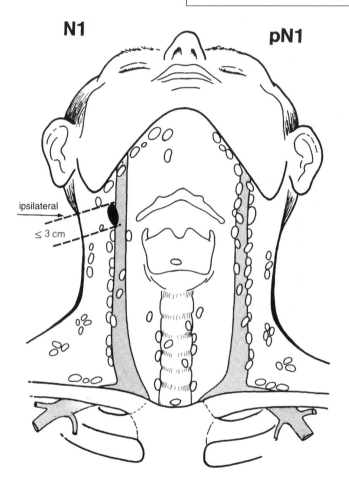

N1

pN1

Any head or neck primary except
nasopharynx and thyroid gland

Fig. 5

ipsilateral

≤ 3 cm

N2/pN2   Metastasis in a single ipsilateral lymph node, more than 3 cm but not more than 6.0 cm in greatest dimension; or in multiple ipsilateral lymph nodes, none more than 6.0 cm in greatest dimension; or in bilateral or contralateral lymph nodes, none more than 6.0 cm in greatest dimension

  N2a/pN2a   Metastasis in a single ipsilateral lymph node, more than 3.0 cm but not more than 6.0 cm in greatest dimension (Fig. 6)

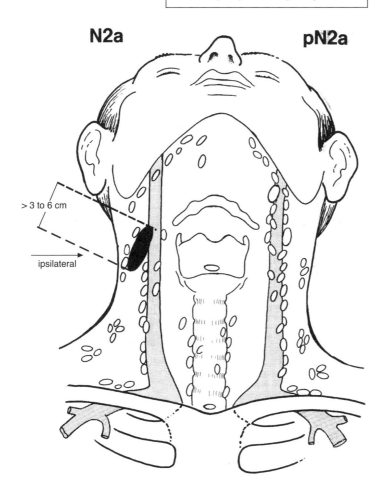

Fig. 6

Any head or neck primary except nasopharynx and thyroid gland

N2a   pN2a

> 3 to 6 cm

ipsilateral

N2b/pN2b   Metastasis in multiple ipsilateral lymph node, none more than 6.0 cm in greatest dimension (Fig. 7)

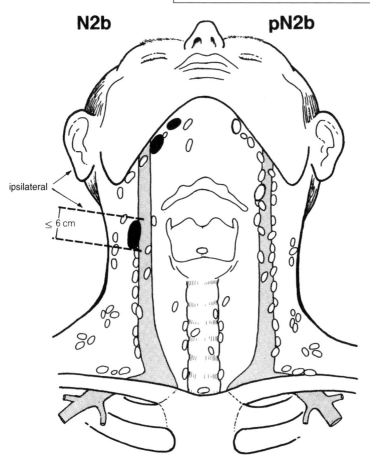

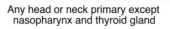

Fig. 7

N2c/pN2c   Metastasis in bilateral or contralateral lymph nodes, none more than 6.0 cm in greatest dimension (Fig. 8)

Fig. 8

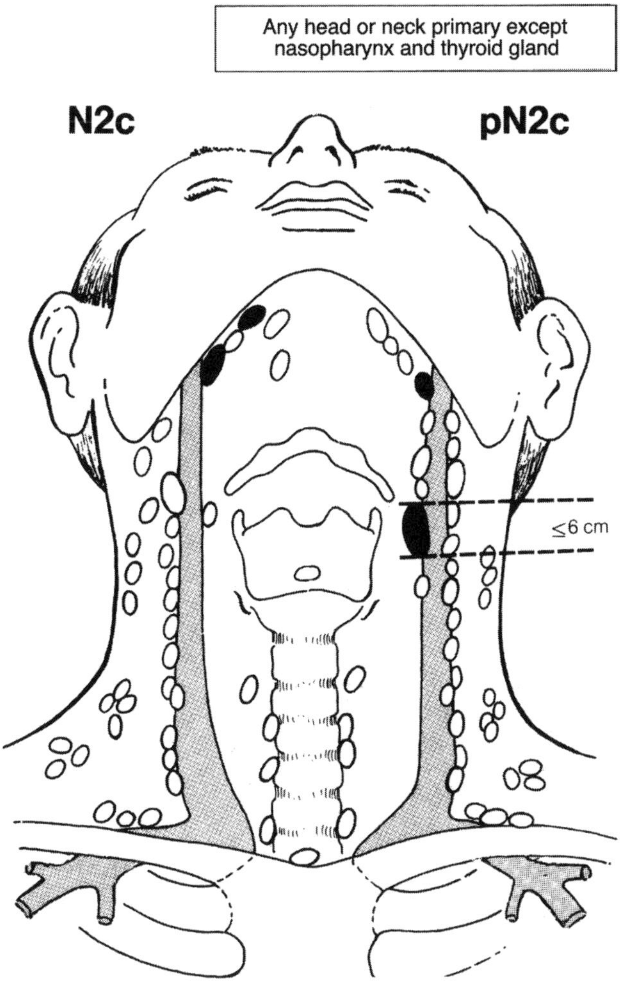

Any head or neck primary except nasopharynx and thyroid gland

N2c   **pN2c**

≤6 cm

N3/pN3   Metastasis in a lymph node, more than 6.0 cm in greatest dimension
          (Fig. 9)

Note
Midline nodes are considered ipsilateral nodes.

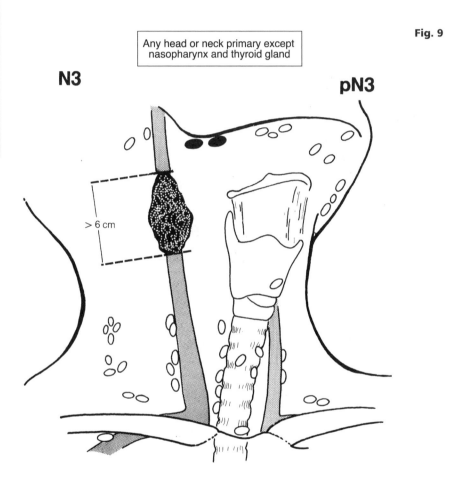

Fig. 9

Any head or neck primary except
nasopharynx and thyroid gland

N3

pN3

> 6 cm

Lip and Oral Cavity (ICD-O C00, C02-C06)

Rules for Classification

The classification applies only to carcinomas of the vermilion surfaces of the lips and of the oral cavity, including those of minor salivary glands. There should be histological confirmation of the disease.

Anatomical Sites and Subsites

Lip (Fig. 10)

1. External upper lip (vermilion border) (C00.0)
2. External lower lip (vermilion border) (C00.1)
3. Commissures (C00.6)

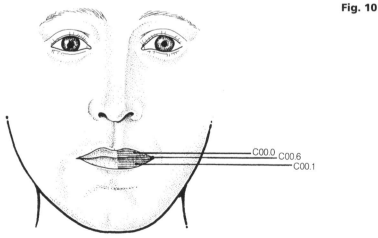

Fig. 10

Oral Cavity (Figs. 11–13)

1. Buccal mucosa
    (i) Mucosa of upper and lower lips (C00.3, 4)
    (ii) Cheek mucosa (C06.0)
    (iii) Retromolar areas (C06.2)
    (iv) Bucco-alveolar sulci, upper and lower (C06.1)
2. Upper alveolus and gingiva (upper gum) (C03.0)
3. Lower alveolus and gingiva (lower gum) (C03.1)
4. Hard palate (C05.0)
5. Tongue
    (i) Dorsal surface and lateral borders anterior to vallate papillae (anterior two-thirds) (C02.0, 1)
    (ii) Inferior (ventral) surface (C02.2)
6. Floor of mouth (C04)

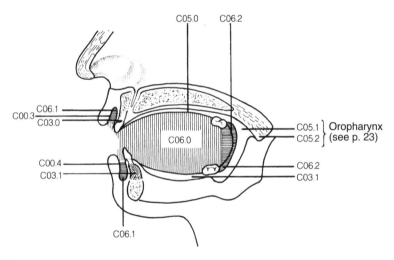

Fig. 11

(see p. 23)

Fig. 12

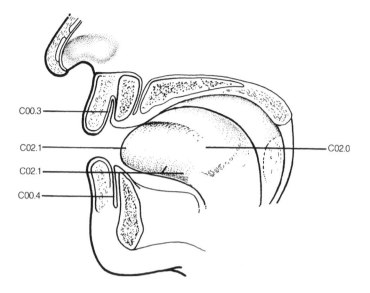

C00.3

C02.1

C02.1

C00.4

C02.0

Fig. 13

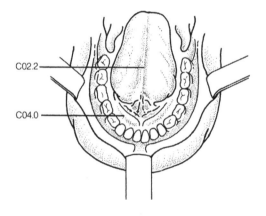

C02.2

C04.0

N—Regional Lymph Nodes

See p. 6.

TN Clinical Classification

T—Primary Tumour

TX   Primary tumour cannot be assessed
T0   No evidence of primary tumour
Tis   Carcinoma in situ

T1   Tumour 2.0 cm or less in greatest dimension (Figs. 14, 15)
T2   Tumour more than 2.0 cm but not more than 4.0 cm in greatest dimension (Figs. 16, 17)
T3   Tumour more than 4.0 cm in greatest dimension (Figs. 18, 19)

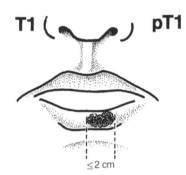

Fig. 14

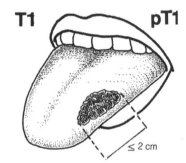

Fig. 15

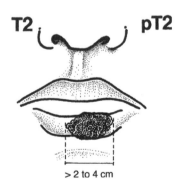

Fig. 16

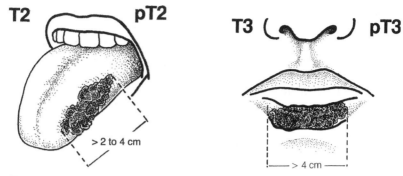

Fig. 17

Fig. 18

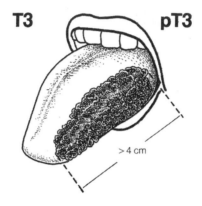

Fig. 19

T4a   *Lip:*   Tumour invades through cortical bone, inferior alveolar nerve, floor
       of mouth, or skin (chin or nose) (Figs. 20, 21)

T4a   *Oral cavity:*   Tumour invades through cortical bone, into deep/extrinsic
       muscle of tongue (genioglossus, hyoglossus, palatoglossus, and styloglossus),
       maxillary sinus, or skin of face (Figs. 22–24)

T4b   *Lip and oral cavity:*   Tumour invades masticator space, pterygoid plates, or
       skull base, or encases internal carotid artery (Fig. 25)

Note

Superficial erosion alone of bone/tooth socket by gingival primary is not sufficient to classify a tumour as
T4a or T4b.

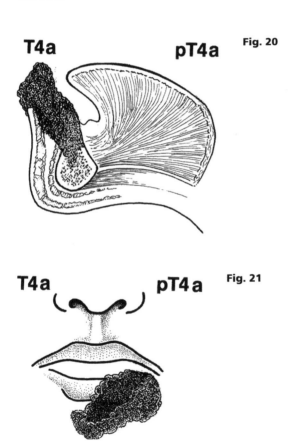

T4a   **pT4a**   **Fig. 20**

T4a   **pT4a**   **Fig. 21**

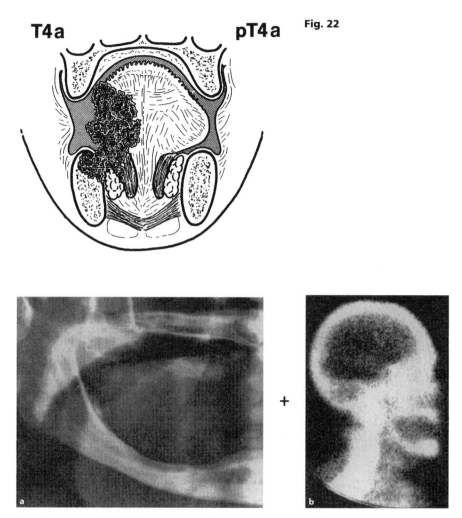

T4a   pT4a   Fig. 22

Fig. 23a. Radiographical suspicion but no evidence of invasion through the cortical bone; the tumour must be classified as non-T4a/b in correspondence with the definitions T1, T2 and T3. **b** Evidence of invasion through cortical bone by uptake, which corresponds with the suspected area in the premolar region of the radiograph shown in **a.** On the basis of the scintigraphic finding the tumour must be classified as T4a.

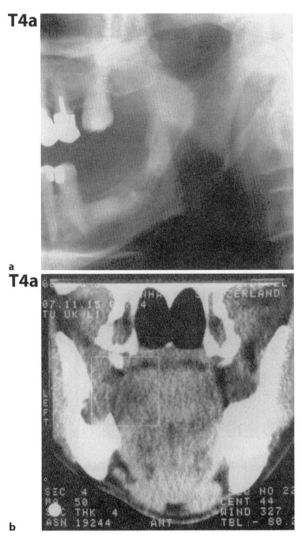

Fig. 24a. Evidence of invasion through cortical bone of the mandibula. **b** CT of case shown in **a.** The carcinoma of the floor of the mouth invades through the cortical bone and into the extrinsic muscle of the tongue (m. hyoglossus).

T4b

pT4b

Fig. 25

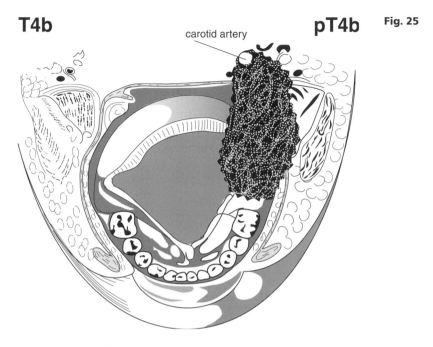

carotid artery

N—Regional Lymph Nodes

See p. 6.

pTN Pathological Classification

The pT and pN categories correspond to the T and N categories.

Summary

Lip, Oral Cavity	
T1	≤2 cm
T2	>2 to 4 cm
T3	>4 cm
T4a	*Lip*: through cortical bone, inferior alveolar nerve, floor of mouth, skin
	Oral cavity: through cortical bone, deep/extrinsic muscle of tongue, maxillary sinus, skin
T4b	Masticator space, pterygoid plates, skull base, internal carotid artery
N1	Ipsilateral single ≤3 cm
N2	(a) Ipsilateral single >3 to 6 cm (b) Ipsilateral multiple ≤6 cm (c) Bilateral, contralateral ≤6 cm
N3	>6 cm

Pharynx (ICD-O C01, C05.1, 2, C09, C10.0, 2, 3, C11-13)

Rules for Classification

The classification applies only to carcinomas. There should be histological confirmation of the disease.

Anatomical Sites and Subsites

Oropharynx (C01, C05.1, 2, C09.0, 1, 9, C10.0, 2, 3) (Figs. 26, 27)

1. Anterior wall (glosso-epiglottic area)
    (i) Base of tongue (posterior to the vallate papillae or posterior third) (C01)
    (ii) Vallecula (C10.0)
2. Lateral wall (C10.2)
    (i) Tonsil (C09.9)
    (ii) Tonsillar fossa (C09.0) and tonsillar (faucial) pillars (C09.1)
    (iii) Glossotonsillar sulci (tonsillar pillars) (C09.1)
3. Posterior wall (C10.3)
4. Superior wall
    (i) Inferior surface of soft palate (C05.1)
    (ii) Uvula (C05.2)

Note
The lingual (anterior) surface of the epiglottis (C10.1) is included with the larynx, suprahyoid epiglottis. (see p. 41).

Fig. 26

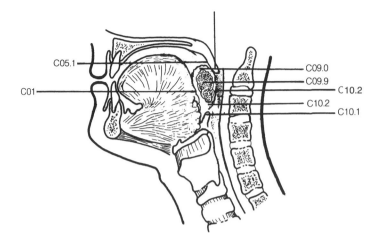

Fig. 27

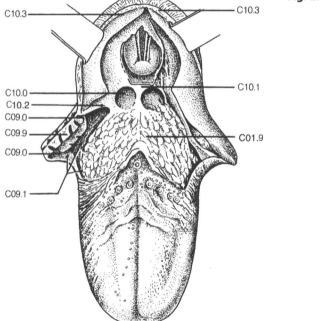

Nasopharynx (C11) (Fig. 28)

1. Postero-superior wall: extends from the level of the junction of the hard and soft palates to the base of the skull (C11.0, 1)
2. Lateral wall: including the fossa of Rosenmüller (C11.2)
3. Inferior wall: consists of the superior surface of the soft palate (C11.3)

Note
The margin of the choanal orifices, including the posterior margin of the nasal septum, is included with the nasal fossa.

Hypopharynx (C12, C13) (Fig. 28)

1. Pharyngo-oesophageal junction (postcricoid area) (C13.0): extends from the level of the arytenoid cartilages and connecting folds to the inferior border of the cricoid cartilage, thus forming the anterior wall of the hypopharynx.
2. Piriform sinus (C12.9): extends from the pharyngo-epiglottic fold to the upper end of the oesophagus. It is bounded laterally by the thyroid cartilage and medially by the hypopharyngeal surface of the aryepiglottic fold (C13.1) and the arytenoid and cricoid cartilages.
3. Posterior pharyngeal wall (C13.2): extends from the superior level of the hyoid bone (or floor of the vallecula) to the level of the inferior border of the cricoid cartilage and from the apex of one piriform sinus to the other.

Regional Lymph Nodes

The regional lymph nodes are the cervical nodes (see p. 6).

The supraclavicular fossa (relevant to classifying nasopharyngeal carcinoma) is the triangular region defined by three points:
(1) the superior margin of the sternal end of the clavicle;
(2) the superior margin of the lateral end of the clavicle;
(3) the point where the neck meets the shoulder.
This includes caudal portions of Levels IV and V (Classification according to Robbins et al.[1]).

---

[1] Robbins KT, Median JE, Wolfe GT, Levine PA, Sesions RB, Pruet CW (1991) Standardizing neck dissection terminology. Official report of the Academy's Committee for Head and Neck Surgery and Oncology. Arch Otolaryngol Head Neck Surg 117:601–605

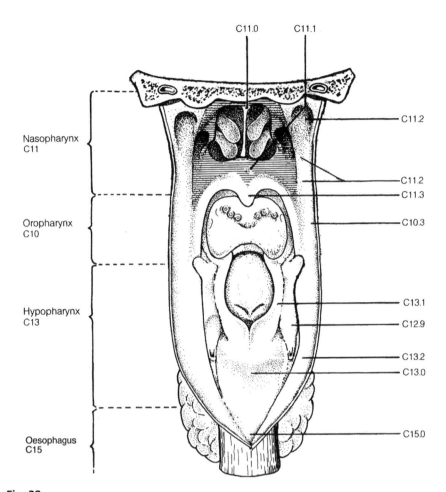

Fig. 28

TN Clinical Classification

T—Primary Tumour

TX   Primary tumour cannot be assessed
T0   No evidence of primary tumour
Tis   Carcinoma in situ

Oropharynx

T1   Tumour 2.0 cm or less in greatest dimension (Fig. 29)
T2   Tumour more than 2.0 cm but not more than 4.0 cm in greatest dimension (Fig. 30)
T3   Tumour more than 4.0 cm in greatest dimension (Fig. 31)

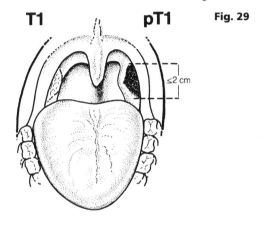

T1   **pT1**   **Fig. 29**

≤2 cm

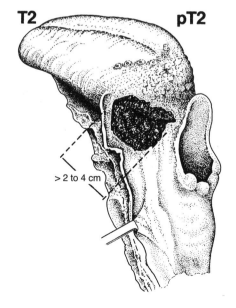

T2   **pT2**   **Fig. 30**

> 2 to 4 cm

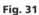

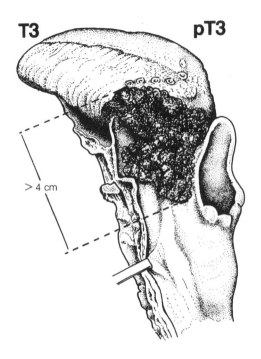

Fig. 31

T4a   Tumour invades any of the following: larynx, deep/extrinsic muscle of
       tongue (genioglossus, hyoglossus, palatoglossus, and styloglossus), medial
       pterygoid, hard palate, and mandible (Fig. 32)

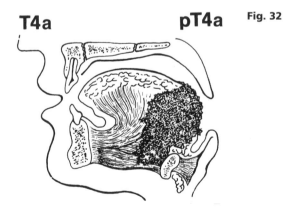

Fig. 32

T4b   Tumour invades any of the following: lateral pterygoid muscle, pterygoid
       plates, lateral nasopharynx, skull base, prevertebral fascia or encases the
       carotid artery (Fig. 33)

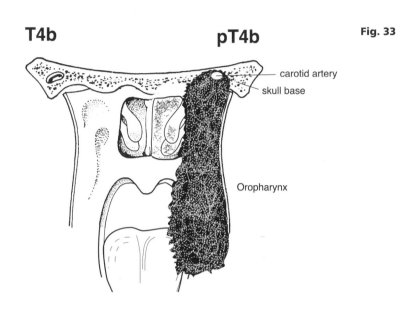

Fig. 33

Nasopharynx

T1   Tumour confined to nasopharynx (Fig. 34)
T2   Tumour extends to soft tissue of oropharynx and/or nasal fossa (Fig. 34)
    T2a   without parapharyngeal extension* (Fig. 35)
    T2b   with parapharyngeal extension* (Fig. 36)
T3   Tumour invades bony structures and/or paranasal sinuses (Fig. 37)
T4   Tumour with intracranial extension and/or involvement of cranial nerves, infratemporal fossa, hypopharynx, orbit, or masticator space (Fig. 38)

Note
* Parapharyngeal extension denotes postero-lateral infiltration of tumour beyond the pharyngo-basilar fascia.

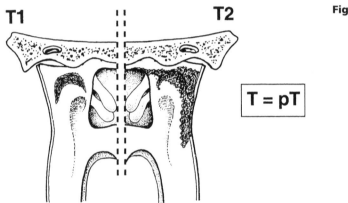

Fig. 34

T1   T2

T = pT

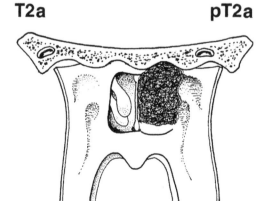

Fig. 35

T2a   pT2a

T2b   **pT2b**   **Fig. 36**

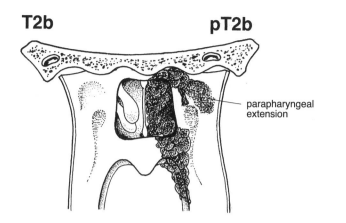

parapharyngeal
extension

T3   **pT3**   **Fig. 37**

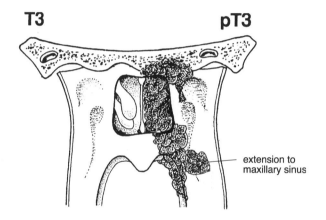

extension to
maxillary sinus

T4   **pT4**   **Fig. 38**

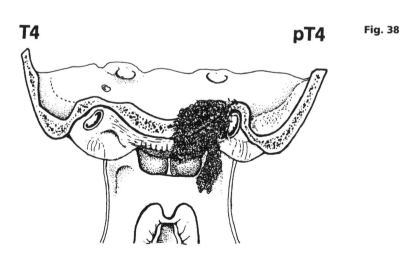

Hypopharynx

T1   Tumour limited to one subsite of hypopharynx (see p. 24–25) and 2.0 cm or less in greatest dimension (Figs. 39–41)

T2   Tumour invades more than one subsite of hypopharynx or an adjacent site, or measures more than 2.0 cm but not more than 4.0 cm in greatest dimension, *without* fixation of hemilarynx (Figs. 42–46)

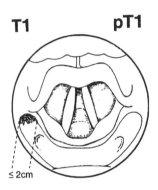

Fig. 39. Involvement of the piriform sinus (C12.9)

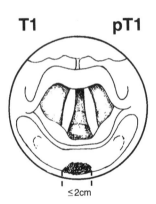

Fig. 40. Involvement of the posterior wall (C13.2)

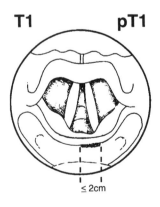

Fig. 41. Involvement of the post-cricoid area (C13.0)

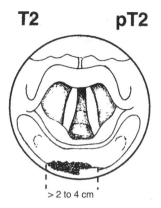

Fig. 42. Involvement of the posterior wall of the hypopharynx (C13.2)

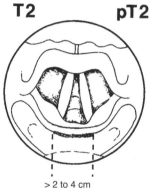

Fig. 43. Involvement of the postcricoid area (C13.0)

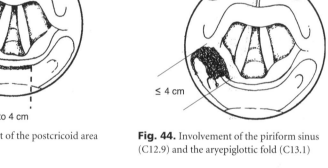

Fig. 44. Involvement of the piriform sinus (C12.9) and the aryepiglottic fold (C13.1)

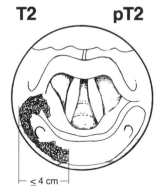

Fig. 45. Involvement of the piriform sinus (C12.9) and the posterior wall of the hypopharynx (C13.2)

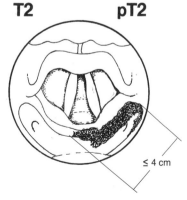

Fig. 46. Involvement of the piriform sinus (C12.9) and the postcricoid area (C13.0)

T3   Tumour measures more than 4.0 cm in greatest dimension, or *with* fixation
      of hemilarynx (Figs. 47–49)

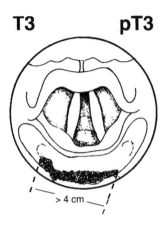

Fig. 47. Involvement of the posterior wall of the hypopharynx (C13.2)

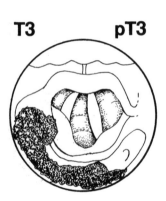

Fig. 48. Invasion of the piriform sinus (C12.9), the aryepiglottic fold (C13.1) and the posterior wall of the hypopharynx (C13.2) with fixation of the hemilarynx

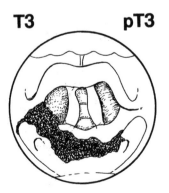

Fig. 49. Invasion of the piriform sinus (C12.9) and postcricoid area (C13.0) with fixation of the hemilarynx

T4a   Tumour invades any of the following: thyroid/cricoid cartilage, hyoid bone, thyroid gland, oesophagus, central compartment soft tissue (Figs. 50–51)

T4b   Tumour invades prevertebral fascia (Fig. 52), encases carotid artery, or invades mediastinal structures

Note
* Central compartment soft tissue includes prelaryngeal strap muscles and subcutaneous fat.

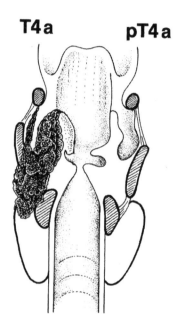

T4a   **pT4a**

Fig. 50. Tumour invasion of the piriform sinus involving the thyroid and cricoid cartilage

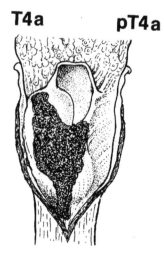

T4a   **pT4a**

Fig. 51. Invasion of adjacent oesophagus

T4b

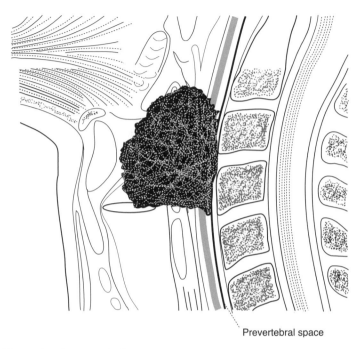

Prevertebral space

Fig. 52. Tumour invades prevertebral space

Oro- and Hypopharynx

N—Regional Lymph Nodes

See p. 6/7.

Nasopharynx

N—Regional Lymph Nodes

NX   Regional lymph nodes cannot be assessed
N0   No regional lymph node metastasis

N1   Unilateral metastasis in lymph node(s), 6.0 cm or less in greatest dimension, above supraclavicular fossa (Fig. 53)

Note
Midline nodes are considered ipsilateral nodes.

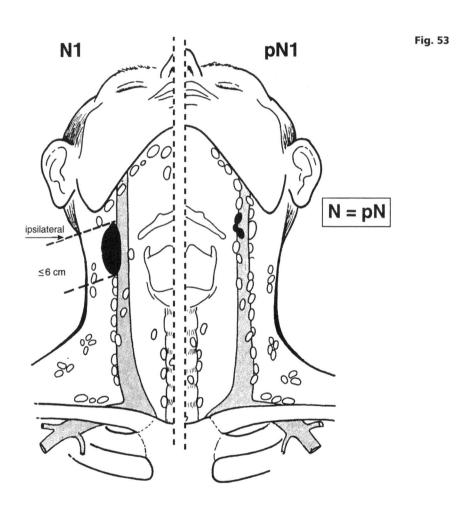

Fig. 53

N2   Bilateral metastasis in lymph node(s), 6.0 cm or less in greatest dimension, above supraclavicular fossa (Fig. 54)

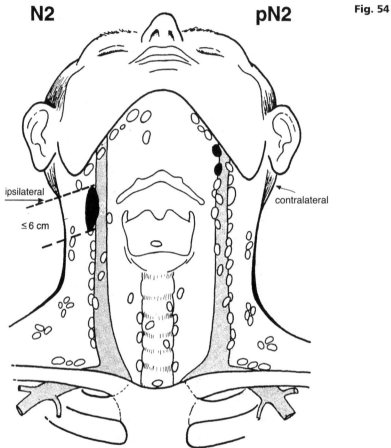

N2   **pN2**   **Fig. 54**

ipsilateral

≤ 6 cm

contralateral

N3   Metastasis in lymph node(s) greater than 6.0 cm in dimension or in the supraclavicular fossa

     N3a   greater than 6.0 cm in dimension

     N3b   in the supraclavicular fossa

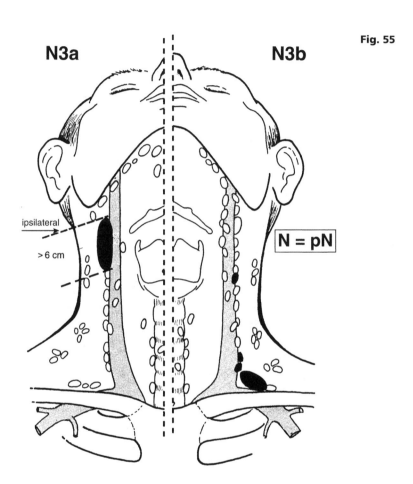

Fig. 55

pTN Pathological Classification

The pT and pN categories correspond to the T and N categories.

Summary

Pharynx	
	Oropharynx
T1	≤2 cm
T2	>2 to 4 cm
T3	>4 cm
T4a	Larynx, deep/extrinsic muscle of tongue, medial pterygoid, hard palate, mandible
T4b	Lateral pterygoid muscle, pterygoid plates, lateral nasopharynx, skull base, prevertebral fascia, carotid artery
	Hypopharynx
T1	≤2 cm and limited to one subsite
T2	>2 to 4 cm or more than one subsite
T3	>4 cm or with hemilarynx fixation
T4a	Thyroid/cricoid cartilage, hyoid bone, thyroid gland, oesophagus, central compartment soft tissue
T4b	Prevertebral fascia, carotid artery, mediastinal structures
	Oropharynx and Hypopharynx
N1	Ipsilateral single ≤3 cm
N2	(a) Ipsilateral single >3 to 6 cm (b) Ipsilateral multiple ≤6 cm (c) Bilateral, contralateral ≤6 cm
N3	>6 cm

Nasopharynx	
T1	Nasopharynx
T2	Soft tissue
T2a	Oropharynx/nasal cavity without parapharyngeal extension
T2b	Tumour with parapharyngeal extension
T3	Bony structures, paranasal sinuses
T4	Intracranial, cranial nerves, infratemporal fossa, hypopharynx, orbit, masticator space
N1	Unilateral node(s) ≤6 cm, above supraclavicular fossa
N2	Bilateral node(s) ≤6 cm, above supraclavicular fossa
N3	(a) >6 cm (b) in supraclavicular fossa

Pharynx

Larynx (ICD-O C32.0, 1, 2, C10.1)

Rules for Classification

The classification applies only to carcinomas. There should be histological confirmation of the disease.

Anatomical Sites and Subsites

(Figs. 26, 27, p. 24, and Figs. 56, 57)

Supraglottis (C32.1)

(i) Suprahyoid epiglottis [including tip, lingual (anterior) (C10.1), and laryngeal surfaces]	} Epilarynx (including marginal zone)
(ii) Aryepiglottic fold, laryngeal aspect	
(iii) Arytenoid	
(iv) Infrahyoid epiglottis	} Supraglottis (excluding epilarynx)
(v) Ventricular bands (false cords)	

Glottis (C32.0)

(i) Vocal cords
(ii) Anterior commissure
(iii) Posterior commissure

Subglottis (C32.2)

Regional Lymph Nodes

See p. 6/7.

Larynx

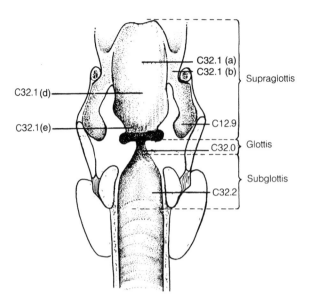

Fig. 56

C32.1 (a)
C32.1 (b)
Supraglottis
C32.1 (d)
C32.1(e)
C12.9
C32.0 } Glottis
Subglottis
C32.2

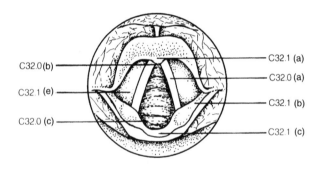

Fig. 57

C32.0(b)
C32.1 (e)
C32.0 (c)
C32.1 (a)
C32.0 (a)
C32.1 (b)
C32.1 (c)

TN Clinical Classification

T—Primary Tumour

TX   Primary tumour cannot be assessed
T0   No evidence of primary tumour
Tis   Carcinoma in situ

Supraglottis

T1   Tumour limited to one subsite of supraglottis with normal vocal cord mobility
(Figs. 58a, b, 59a, b)

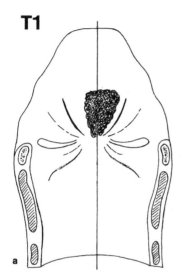
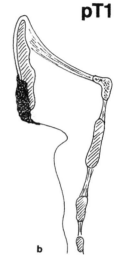

Fig. 58a, b. Involvement of the epiglottis

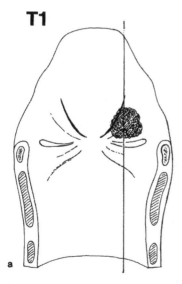
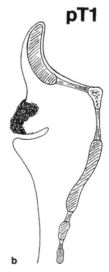

Fig. 59a, b. Involvement of the false cord

T2   Tumour invades mucosa of more than one adjacent subsite of supraglottis or glottis or region outside the supraglottis (e.g., mucosa of base of tongue, vallecula, medial wall of piriform sinus) without fixation of the larynx (Figs. 60a, b, 61a, b)

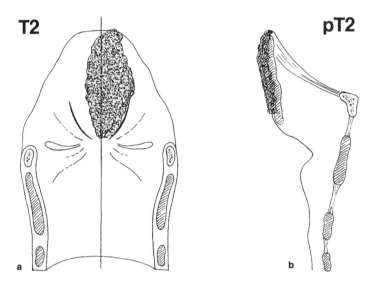

Fig. 60a, b. Involvement of the suprahyoid and the mucosa of the infrahyoid epiglottis

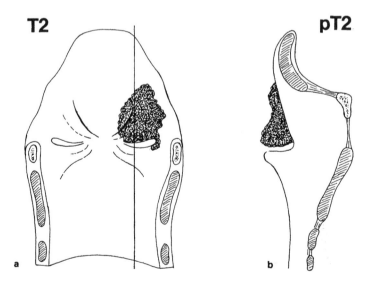

Fig. 61a, b. Involvement of the false cord and the epiglottis

T3   Tumour limited to larynx with vocal cord fixation and/or invades any of the following: postcricoid area, pre-epiglottic tissues, paraglottic space, and/or with minor thyroid cartilage erosion (e.g., inner cortex) (Figs. 62a, b, 63a, b)

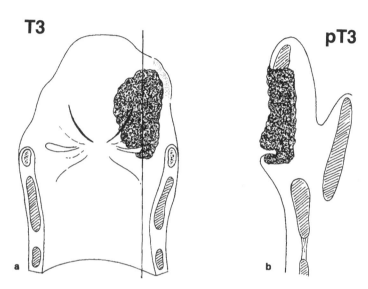

Fig. 62a, b. Involvement of supraglottis and vocal cord with cord fixation

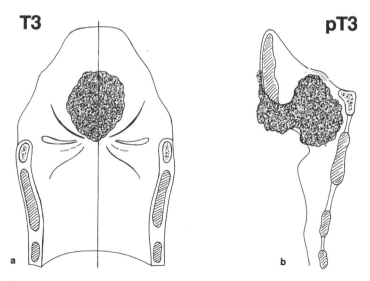

Fig. 63a, b. Invasion of the pre-epiglottic tissues with vocal cord fixation

T4a   Tumour invades through thyroid cartilage, and/or invades tissues beyond the
       larynx, e.g., trachea, soft tissues of the neck including deep/extrinsic muscle
       of tongue (genioglossus, hyoglossus, palatoglossus, and styloglossus), strap
       muscles, thyroid, oesophagus (Fig. 64a, b)

T4b   Tumour invades prevertebral space, mediastinal structures, or encases carotid
       artery (Fig. 52)

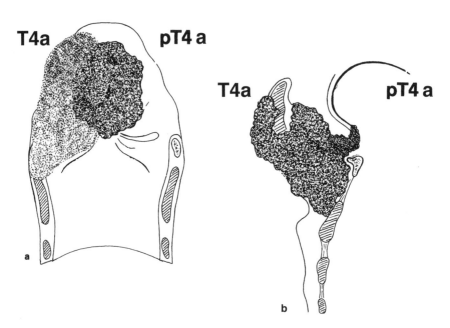

Fig. 64a, b. Invasion beyond the larynx (vallecula and base of tongue) and soft tissues of the neck
(pre-larynx)

Glottis

T1 Tumour limited to vocal cord(s) (may involve anterior or posterior commissure) with normal mobility (Fig. 65a)

    T1a   Tumour limited to one vocal cord (Fig. 65b)

    T1b   Tumour involves both vocal cords (Fig. 65c)

T2 Tumour extends to supraglottis and/or subglottis, and/or with impaired vocal cord mobility (Fig. 66a, b)

T3 Tumour limited to larynx with vocal cord fixation
and/or invades paraglottic space, and/or with minor thyroid cartilage erosion (e.g., inner cortex) (Fig. 67a, b)

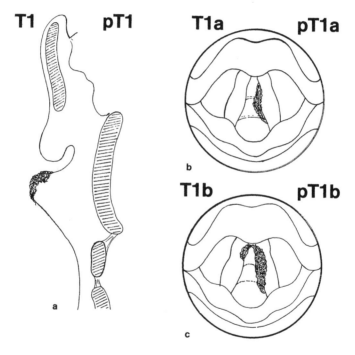

Fig. 65a–c. Tumour limited to vocal cord (**a, b**). **c** Tumour limited to vocal cords with invasion of the anterior commissure

Larynx

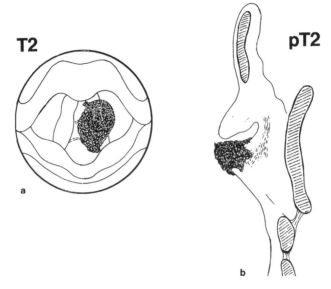

Fig. 66a, b. Tumour extends to supraglottis with impaired vocal cord mobility by invasion of the superficial m. vocalis

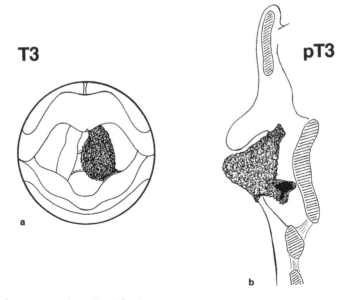

Fig. 67a, b. Tumour with vocal cord fixation

T4a   Tumour invades through thyroid cartilage or other tissues beyond the larynx,
       e.g., trachea, soft tissues of neck including deep/extrinsic muscle of tongue
       (genioglossus, hyoglossus, palatoglossus, and styloglossus), strap muscles,
       thyroid, oesophagus (Fig. 68a, b)
T4b   Tumour invades prevertebral space, mediastinal structures, or encases carotid
       artery (Fig. 69)

T4a

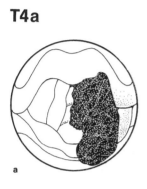

pT4a

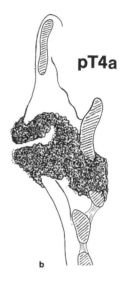

Fig. 68a, b.
Tumour invades
beyond the larynx (**a**)
and invades thyroid
cartilage (**b**)

T4b

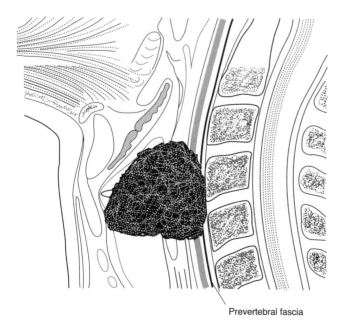

Fig. 69. Tumour
invades prevertebral
space

Prevertebral fascia

Subglottis

T1   Tumour limited to subglottis (Fig. 70a, b)
T2   Tumour extends to vocal cord(s) with normal or impaired mobility
      (Fig. 71a, b)

Fig. 70

T1

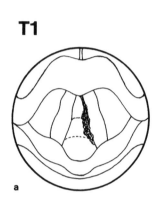

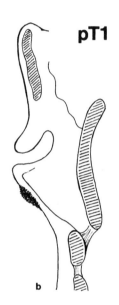

pT1

Fig. 71

T2

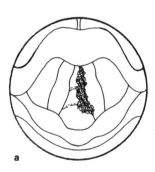

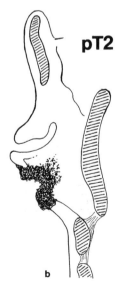

pT2

T3   Tumour limited to larynx with vocal cord fixation (Fig. 72)

T4a   Tumour invades through cricoid or thyroid cartilage and/or invades into other tissues beyond the larynx, e.g., trachea, soft tissues of neck including deep/extrinsic muscle of tongue (genioglossus, hyoglossus, palatoglossus, and styloglossus), strap muscles, thyroid, oesophagus (Fig. 73)

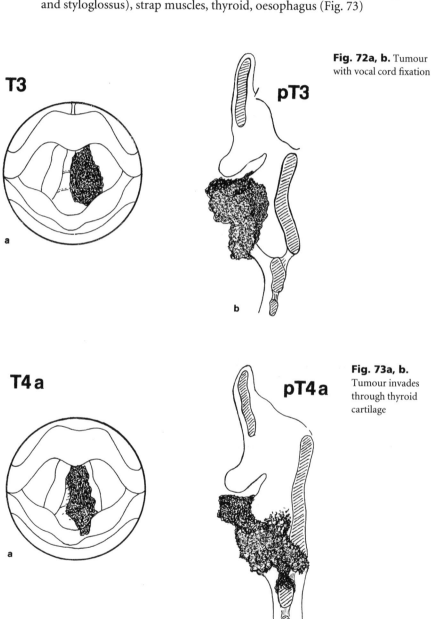

T3

pT3

Fig. 72a, b. Tumour with vocal cord fixation

T4a

pT4a

Fig. 73a, b. Tumour invades through thyroid cartilage

T4b   Tumour invades prevertebral space, mediastinal structures, or encases carotid artery (Fig. 74)

T4b

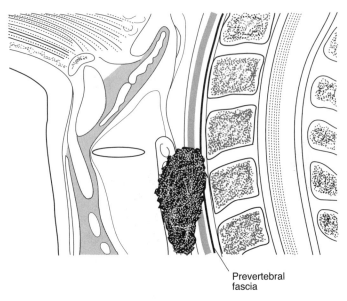

Prevertebral
fascia

Fig. 74. Tumour invades prevertebral space

N—Regional Lymph Nodes

See p. 6/7.

pTN Pathological Classification

The pT and pN categories correspond to the T and N categories.

Summary

Larynx	
	Supraglottis
T1	One subsite, normal mobility
T2	Mucosa of more than one adjacent subsite of supraglottis or glottis or adjacent region outside the supraglottis; without fixation
T3	Cord fixation or invades postcricoid area, pre-epiglottic tissues, paraglottic space, thyroid cartilage erosion
T4a	Through thyroid cartilage; trachea, soft tissues of neck: deep/extrinsic muscle of tongue, strap muscles, thyroid, oesophagus
T4b	Prevertebral space, mediastinal structures, carotid artery
	Glottis
T1	Limited to vocal cord(s), normal mobility (a) one cord (b) both cords
T2	Supraglottis, subglottis, impaired cord mobility
T3	Cord fixation, paraglottic space, thyroid cartilage erosion
T4a	Through thyroid cartilage; trachea, soft tissues of neck: deep/extrinsic muscle of tongue, strap muscles, thyroid, oesophagus
T4b	Prevertebral space, mediastinal structures, carotid artery
	Subglottis
T1	Limited to subglottis
T2	Extends to vocal cord(s) with normal/impaired mobility
T3	Cord fixation
T4a	Through cricoid or thyroid cartilage; trachea, deep/extrinsic muscle of tongue, strap muscles, thyroid, oesophagus
T4b	Prevertebral space, mediastinal structures, carotid artery
	All Sites
N1	Ipsilateral single ≤3 cm
N2	(a) Ipsilateral single >3 to 6 cm (b) Ipsilateral multiple ≤6 cm (c) Bilateral, contralateral ≤6 cm
N3	>6 cm

Nasal Cavity and Paranasal Sinuses (ICD-C30.0, C31.0, 1)

Rules for Classification

The classification applies only to carcinomas. There should be histological confirmation of the disease.

Anatomical Sites and Subsites

1. ***Nasal Cavity (C30.0)*** (Fig. 75)
   - Septum
   - Floor
   - Lateral wall
   - Vestibule
2. ***Maxillary Sinus (C31.0)*** (Fig. 76)
3. ***Ethmoid Sinus (C31.1)*** (Fig. 76)
   - Left
   - Right

Regional Lymph Nodes

See p. 6/7.

Fig. 75

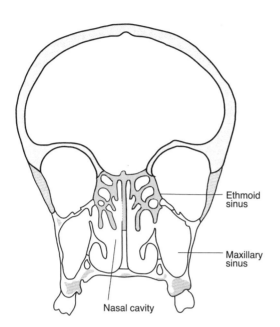

Ethmoid
sinus

Maxillary
sinus

Nasal cavity

Fig. 76

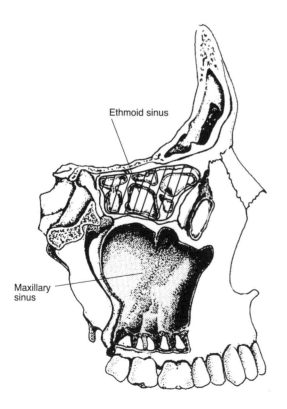

Ethmoid sinus

Maxillary
sinus

TN Clinical Classification

T—Primary Tumour

TX   Primary tumour cannot be assessed
T0   No evidence of primary tumour
Tis   Carcinoma in situ

Maxillary Sinus

T1   Tumour limited to the antral mucosa with no erosion or destruction of bone
        (Fig. 77)
T2   Tumour causing bone erosion or destruction including extension into hard
        palate and/or middle nasal meatus, except extension to posterior wall of
        maxillary sinus and pterygoid plates (Fig. 78)

Fig. 77

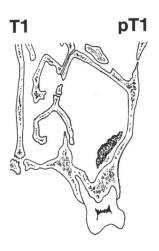

T1   pT1

Fig. 78

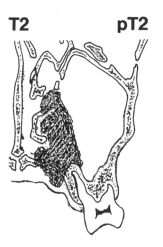

T2   pT2

T3   Tumour invades any of the following: bone of posterior wall of maxillary sinus, subcutaneous tissues, floor or medial wall of orbit pterygoid fossa, ethmoid sinuses (Figs. 79, 80)

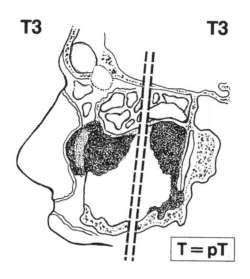

Fig. 79

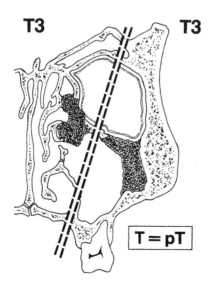

Fig. 80. Tumour of the maxillary sinus with invasion of the medial wall of the orbit and of ethmoid sinus

T4a   Tumour invades any of the following: anterior orbital contents, skin of cheek, pterygoid plates, infratemporal fossa, cribriform plate, sphenoid or frontal sinuses (Figs. 81, 82)

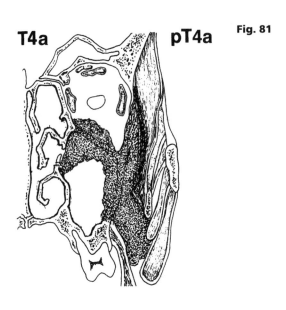

T4a   **pT4a**   Fig. 81

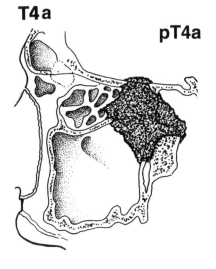

T4a   Fig. 82

pT4a

T4b   Tumour invades any of the following: orbital apex, dura, brain, middle cranial fossa, cranial nerves other than maxillary division of trigeminal nerve (V2), nasopharynx, clivus (Fig. 83)

T4b   pT4b   Fig. 83

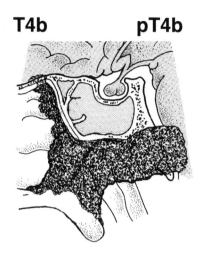

Nasal Cavity and Ethmoid Sinus

T1   Tumour restricted to one subsite of nasal cavity or ethmoid sinus, with or
       without bony invasion (Figs. 84, 85)

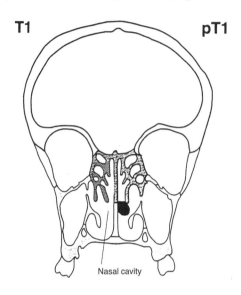

Fig. 84

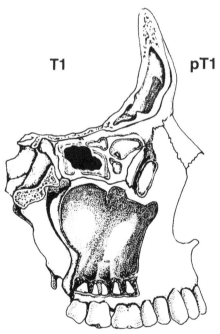

Fig. 85

T2   Tumour involves two subsites in a single site or extends to involve an adjacent site within the nasoethmoidal complex, with or without bony invasion (Fig. 86)

T3   Tumour extends to invade the medial wall or floor of the orbit, maxillary sinus, palate, or cribriform plate (Fig. 87)

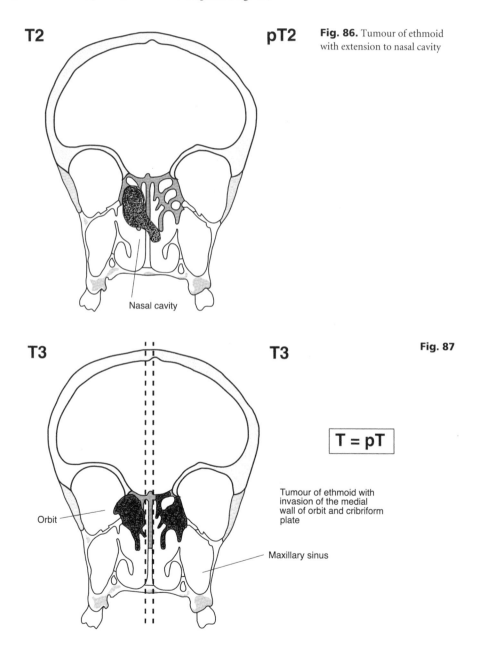

Fig. 86. Tumour of ethmoid with extension to nasal cavity

Fig. 87

T = pT

Tumour of ethmoid with invasion of the medial wall of orbit and cribriform plate

T4a   Tumour invades any of the following: anterior orbital contents, skin of
      nose or cheek, minimal extension to anterior cranial fossa, pterygoid plates,
      sphenoid or frontal sinuses (Fig. 88)

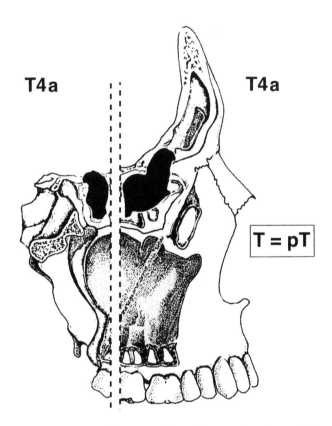

Fig. 88. Tumor of ethmoid sinus with invasion of frontal sinuses and anterior cranial fossa

T4b   Tumour invades any of the following: orbital apex, dura, brain, middle cranial fossa, cranial nerves other than V2, nasopharynx, clivus (Fig. 89)

Fig. 89

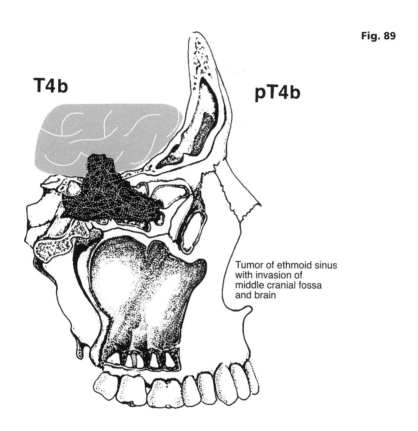

T4b

pT4b

Tumor of ethmoid sinus with invasion of middle cranial fossa and brain

N—Regional Lymph Nodes

See p. 6/7.

pTN Pathological Classification

The pT and pN categories correspond to the T and N categories.

Summary

Nasal Cavity and Paranasal Sinuses	
	Maxillary Sinus
T1	Mucosa
T2	Bone erosion/destruction, hard palate, middle nasal meatus
T3	Posterior bony wall maxillary sinus, subcutaneous tissues, floor/medial wall of orbit, pterygoid fossa, ethmoid sinus
T4a	Anterior orbit, cheek skin, pterygoid plates, infratemporal fossa, cribriform plate, sphenoid/frontal sinus
T4b	Orbital apex, dura, brain, middle cranial fossa, cranial nerves other than V2, nasopharynx, clivus
	Nasal Cavity and Ethmoid Sinus
T1	One subsite
T2	Two subsites or adjacent nasoethmoidal site
T3	Medial wall/floor orbit, maxillary sinus, palate, cribriform plate
T4a	Anterior orbit, skin of nose/cheek, anterior cranial fossa (minimal), pterygoid plates, sphenoid/frontal sinuses
T4b	Orbital apex, dura, brain, middle cranial fossa, cranial nerves other than V2, nasopharynx, clivus
	All Sites
N1	Ipsilateral single ≤3 cm
N2	(a) Ipsilateral single >3 to 6 cm (b) Ipsilateral multiple ≤6 cm (c) Bilateral, contralateral ≤6 cm
N3	>6 cm

Salivary Glands (ICD-O C07, C08)

Rules for Classification

The classification applies only to carcinomas of the major salivary glands: parotid (C07.9), submandibular (submaxillary) (C08.0), and sublingual (C08.1) glands. Tumours arising in minor salivary glands (mucus-secreting glands in the lining membrane of the upper aerodigestive tract) are not included in this classification but at their anatomic site of origin, e.g., lip. There should be histological confirmation of the disease.

Regional Lymph Nodes

The regional lymph nodes are the cervical nodes (see p. 6/7).

TNM Clinical Classification

T—Primary Tumour

TX   Primary tumour cannot be assessed
T0   No evidence of primary tumour

T1   Tumour 2.0 cm or less in greatest dimension without extraparenchymal extension* (Fig. 90)
T2   Tumour more than 2.0 cm but not more than 4.0 cm in greatest dimension without extraparenchymal extension* (Fig. 91)

Note

* Extraparenchymal extension is clinical or macroscopic evidence of invasion of soft tissues or nerve, except those listed under T4a and T4b. Microscopic evidence alone does not constitute extraparenchymal extension for classification purposes.

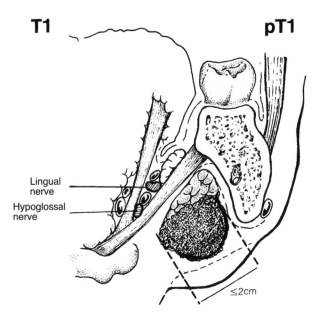

Fig. 90. Classification determined clinically on the basis of absence of paralysis or macroscopically on the basis of no extraparenchymal extension. Frontal section through the premolar region

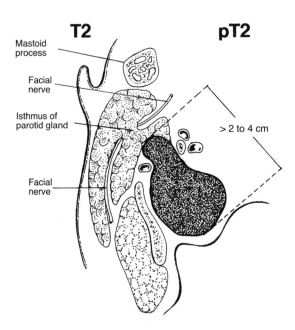

Fig. 91. Horizontal section through the parotid gland showing its supposed division into superficial and deep lobes

T3   Tumour more than 4 cm and/or tumour having extraparenchymal extension*
(Figs. 92, 93)

Note
See p. 65.

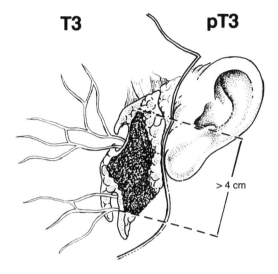

Fig. 92. Tumour more than 4 cm without extraparenchymal extension

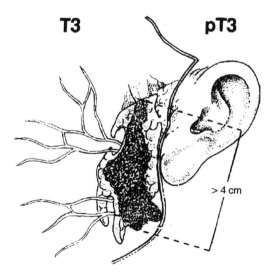

Fig. 93. Tumour more than 4 cm with extraparenchymal extension

T4a   Tumour invades skin, mandible, ear canal, or facial nerve (Fig. 94)

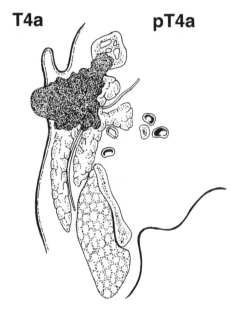

Fig. 94. Invasion of the facial nerve and of skin

T4b   Tumour invades base of skull, pterygoid plates, or encases carotid artery (Fig. 95)

pT4b

Fig. 95

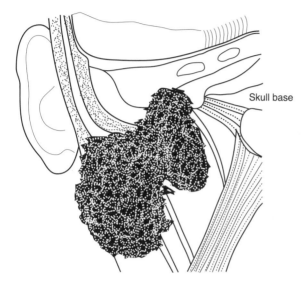

Skull base

N—Regional Lymph Nodes

See p. 6/7.

pTN Pathological Classification

The pT and pN categories correspond to the T and N categories.

Summary

Salivary Glands	
T1	≤ 2 cm, without extraparenchymal extension
T2	>2 to 4 cm, without extraparenchymal extension
T3	>4 cm and/or extraparenchymal extension,
T4a	Skin, mandible, ear canal, facial nerve
T4b	Skull, pterygoid plates, carotid artery
N1	Ipsilateral single ≤3 cm
N2	(a) Ipsilateral single >3 to 6 cm (b) Ipsilateral multiple ≤6 cm (c) Bilateral, contralateral ≤6 cm
N3	>6 cm

Thyroid Gland (ICD-O C73) (FIG. 96)

Rules for Classification

The classification applies only to carcinomas. There should be microscopic confirmation of the disease and division of cases by histological type.

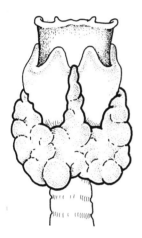

Fig. 96

Regional Lymph Nodes (Fig. 97)

The regional lymph nodes are the cervical and upper/superior mediastinal nodes.

Fig. 97

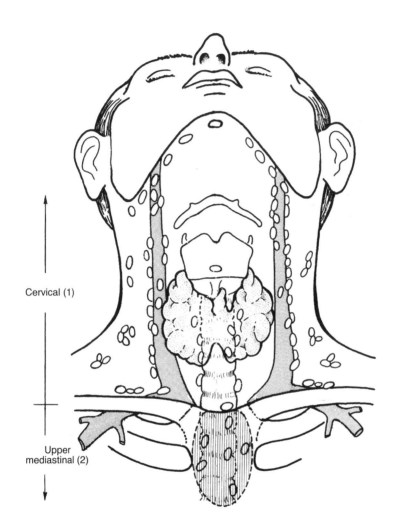

Cervical (1)

Upper
mediastinal (2)

TN Clinical Classification

T—Primary Tumour

TX   Primary tumour cannot be assessed
T0   No evidence of primary tumour

All histological types except undifferentiated carcinoma
T1   Tumour 2 cm or less in greatest dimension, limited to the thyroid (Fig. 98)
T2   Tumour more than 2 cm but not more than 4 cm in greatest dimension, limited to the thyroid (Fig. 99)
T3   Tumour more than 4 cm in greatest dimension, limited to the thyroid or any tumour with minimal extrathyroidal extension (e.g., extension to sternothyroid muscle or perithyroid soft tissues) (Figs. 100, 101)
T4a   Tumour extends beyond the thyroid capsule and invades any of the following: subcutaneous soft tissues, larynx, trachea, oesophagus, recurrent laryngeal nerve (Fig. 102)
T4b   Tumour invades prevertebral fascia, mediastinal vessels or encases carotid artery (Fig. 103)

Undifferentiated carcinoma (all are classified as T4)
T4a[1]   Tumour (any size) limited to the thyroid, considered surgically resectable
T4b[1]   Tumour (any size) extends beyond the thyroid capsule, considered surgically unresectable

Note
Multifocal tumours should be designated (m) (the largest determines the classification), e.g., T2(m).

Thyroid Gland

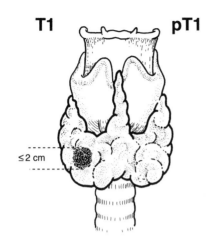

Fig. 98

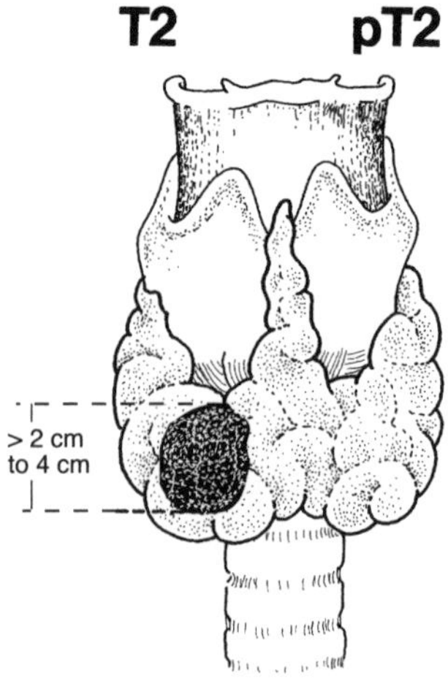

Fig. 99

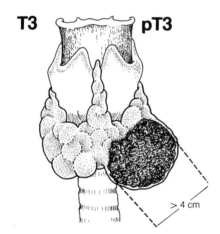

Fig. 100

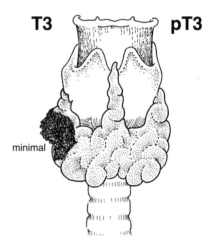

Fig. 101

T4a   pT4a   Fig. 102

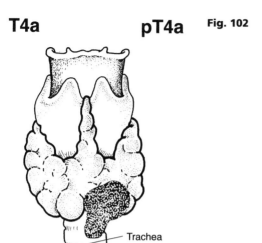

Trachea

T4b   pT4b   Fig. 103

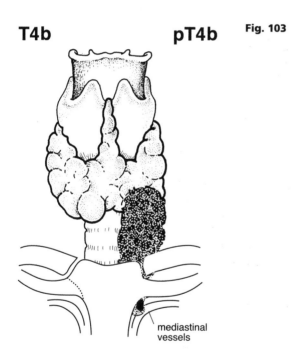

mediastinal
vessels

N—Regional Lymph Nodes

NX   Regional lymph nodes cannot be assessed
N0   No regional lymph node metastasis
N1a   Metastasis in Level VI (pretracheal, paratracheal, including prelaryngeal and
        Delphian lymph node(s)) (see p. 6) (Fig. 104)
N1b   Metastasis in other unilateral, bilateral, or contralateral cervical or upper/
        superior mediastinal lymph node(s) (Fig. 105)

pTN Pathological Classification

The pT and pN categories correspond to the T and N categories.

pN0 Histological examination of a selective neck dissection specimen will ordinarily
include 6 or more lymph nodes.
If the examined lymph nodes are negative, but the number ordinarily resected is not
met, classify as pN0.

N1a   pN1a   Fig. 104

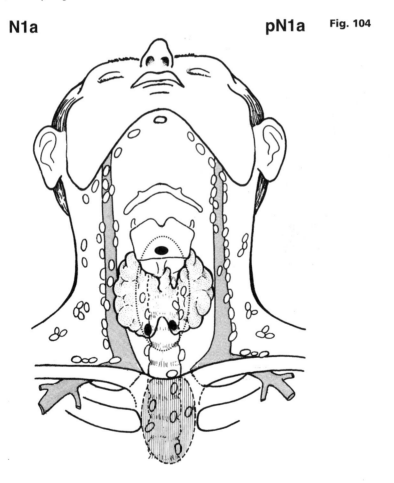

Fig. 105

N1b

pN1b

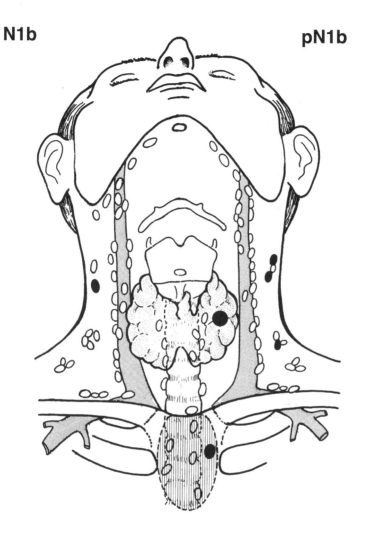

Summary

Thyroid Gland	
	Papillary, follicular and medullary carcinoma
T1	≤2 cm intrathyroidal
T2	>2 to 4 cm intrathyroidal
T3	>4 cm or minimal extension
T4a	Subcutaneous, larynx, trachea, oesophagus, recurrent laryngeal nerve
T4b	Prevertebral fascia, mediastinal vessels, carotid artery
	Anaplastic/undifferentiated carcinoma
T4a	Tumour limited to thyroid
T4b	Tumour beyond thyroid capsule
	All types
N1a	Level VI
N1b	Other regional

Digestive System Tumours

Introductory Notes

The following sites are included:

- Oesophagus
- Stomach
- Small Intestine
- Colon and Rectum
- Anal Canal
- Liver
- Gallbladder
- Extrahepatic Bile Ducts
- Ampulla of Vater
- Pancreas (excluding endocrine part)

Regional Lymph Nodes

The number of lymph nodes ordinarily included in a lymphadenectomy specimen is noted at each site.

TNM Atlas: Illustrated Guide to the TNM Classification of Malignant Tumours, Fifth Edition,
edited by Christian Wittekind, Frederick L. Greene, Robert Hutter, Martin Klimpfinger, and Leslie H. Sobin
Copyright © 2005 UICC

Oesophagus (ICD-O C15)

Rules for Classification

The classification applies only to carcinomas. There should be histological confirmation of the disease and division of cases by histological type.

Anatomical Subsites (Fig. 106)

1. **Cervical oesophagus** (C15.0):
   This commences at the lower border of the cricoid cartilage and ends at the thoracic inlet (suprasternal notch), approximately 18.0 cm from the upper incisor teeth.
2. **Intrathoracic oesophagus**
   (i) The upper thoracic portion (C15.3) extending from the thoracic inlet to the level of the tracheal bifurcation, approximately 24 cm from the upper incisor teeth.
   (ii) The mid-thoracic portion (C15.4) is the proximal half of the oesophagus between the tracheal bifurcation and the oesophagogastric junction. The lower level is approximately 32 cm from the upper incisor teeth.
   (iii) The lower thoracic portion (C15.5), approximately 8 cm in length (includes abdominal oesophagus), is the distal half of the oesophagus between the tracheal bifurcation and the oesophagogastric junction. The lower level is approximately 40 cm from the upper incisor teeth.

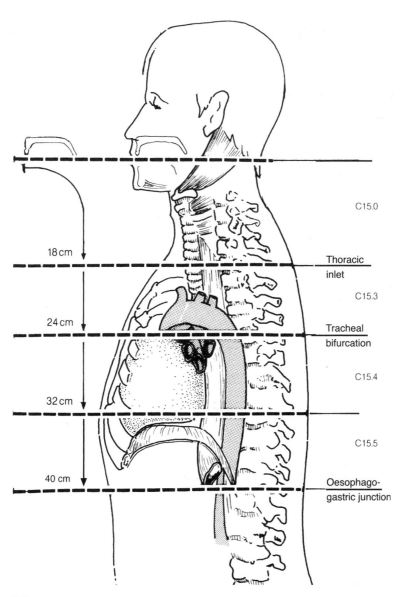

Fig. 106

Regional Lymph Nodes

The regional lymph nodes are as follows (Fig. 107):

Cervical oesophagus:

- Scalene
- Internal jugular
- Upper and lower cervical
- Perioesophageal
- Supraclavicular

Intrathoracic oesophagus—upper, middle, and lower:

- Upper perioesophageal (above the azygos vein)
- Subcarinal
- Lower perioesophageal (below the azygos vein)
- Mediastinal lymph nodes
- Perigastric lymph nodes (except coeliac lymph nodes)

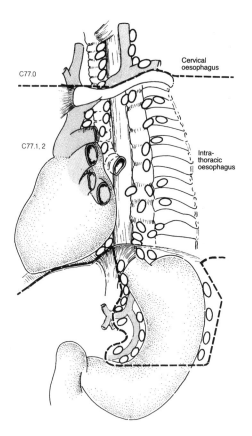

Fig. 107

C77.0

Cervical
oesophagus

C77.1, 2

Intra-
thoracic
oesophagus

TNM Clinical Classification

T—Primary Tumour

TX   Primary tumour cannot be assessed
T0   No evidence of primary tumour
Tis   Carcinoma in situ

T1   Tumour invades lamina propria or submucosa (Fig. 108)
T2   Tumour invades muscularis propria (Fig. 109)

Fig. 108   **Fig. 109**

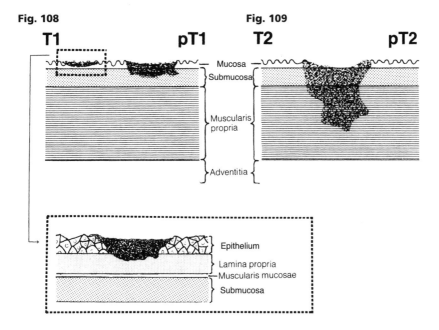

T3   Tumour invades adventitia (Fig. 110)
T4   Tumour invades adjacent structures (Fig. 111)

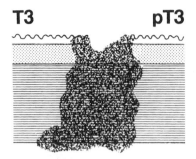

T3   **pT3**   **Fig. 110**

Fig. 111

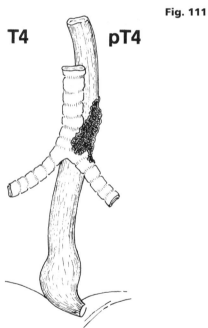

T4   **pT4**

N—Regional Lymph Nodes

NX   Regional lymph nodes cannot be assessed
N0   No regional lymph node metastasis
N1   Regional lymph node metastasis (Figs. 112–115)

Carcinoma of cervical oesophagus

Fig. 112

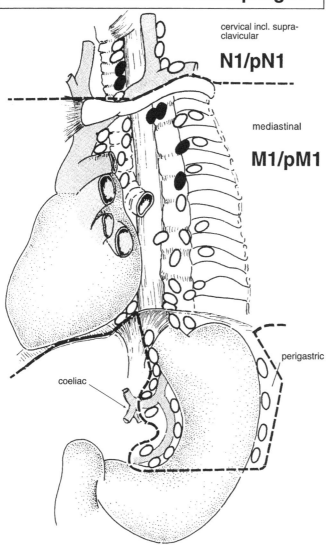

cervical incl. supra-
clavicular

N1/pN1

mediastinal

M1/pM1

perigastric

coeliac

Fig. 113

Carcinoma of upper thoracic oesophagus

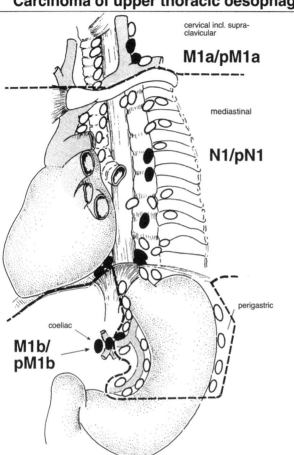

cervical incl. supra-clavicular

M1a/pM1a

mediastinal

N1/pN1

perigastric

coeliac

M1b/ pM1b

Fig. 114

Carcinoma of mid-thoracic oesophagus

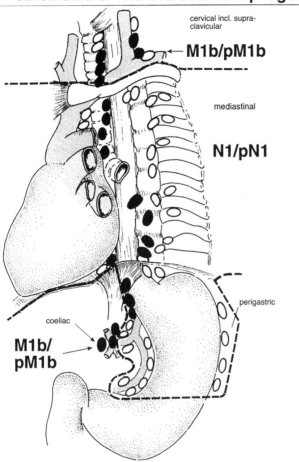

Fig. 115

Carcinoma of lower thoracic oesophagus

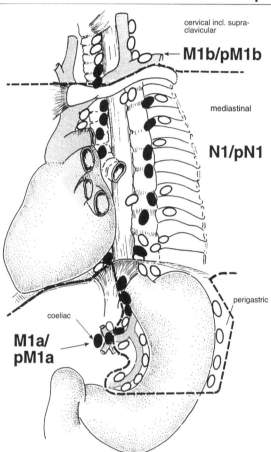

cervical incl. supra-
clavicular

← **M1b/pM1b**

mediastinal

N1/pN1

perigastric

coeliac

**M1a/
pM1a**

Oesophagus

M—Distant Metastasis

MX   Distant metastasis cannot be assessed
M0   No distant metastasis
M1   Distant metastasis

For tumours of lower thoracic oesophagus (Fig. 115)

    M1a   Metastasis in coeliac lymph nodes
    M1b   Other distant metastasis

For tumours of upper thoracic oesophagus (Fig. 113)

    M1a   Metastasis in cervical lymph nodes
    M1b   Other distant metastasis

For tumours of mid-thoracic oesophagus (Fig. 114)

    M1a   Not applicable
    M1b   Non-regional lymph nodes or other distant metastasis

pTNM Pathological Classification

The pT, pN, and pM categories correspond to the T, N, and M categories.

pN0 Histological examination of a mediastinal lymphadenectomy specimen will ordinarily include 6 or more lymph nodes. If the examined lymph nodes are negative, but the number ordinarily resected is not met, classify as pN0.

Summary

Oesophagus	
T1	Lamina propria, submucosa
T2	Muscularis propria
T3	Adventitia
T4	Adjacent structures
N1	Regional
M1	Distant metastasis
	Tumour of *lower thoracic* oesophagus
M1a	Coeliac nodes
M1b	Other distant metastasis
	Tumour of *upper thoracic* oesophagus
M1a	Cervical nodes
M1b	Other distant metastasis
	Tumour of *mid-thoracic* oesophagus
M1b	Distant metastasis including non-regional lymph nodes

Stomach (ICD-O C16)

Rules for Classification

The classification applies only to carcinomas. There should be histological confirmation of the disease.

Anatomical Subsites (Fig. 116)

1. Cardia (gastroesophageal junction) (C16.0)
2. Fundus (C16.1)
3. Corpus (C16.2)
4. Antrum (C16.3) and pylorus (C16.4)

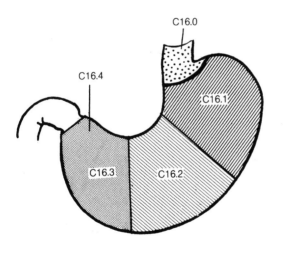

Fig. 116

C16.0

C16.4

C16.1

C16.3

C16.2

Regional Lymph Nodes (Fig. 117,118)

The regional lymph nodes of the stomach are the perigastric nodes along the lesser (1, 3, 5) and greater curvatures (2, 4a, 4b, 6), the nodes along the left gastric (7), common hepatic (8), splenic (11), and coeliac arteries (9), and the hepatoduodenal nodes (12).

The regional lymph nodes of the gastroesophageal junction are the paracardial (1, 2), left gastric (7), coeliac (9), diaphragmatic, and the lower mediastinal paraoesophageal (see p. 76, Fig. 107).

Involvement of other intra-abdominal lymph nodes such as retropancreatic, mesenteric, and para-aortic is classified as distant metastasis.

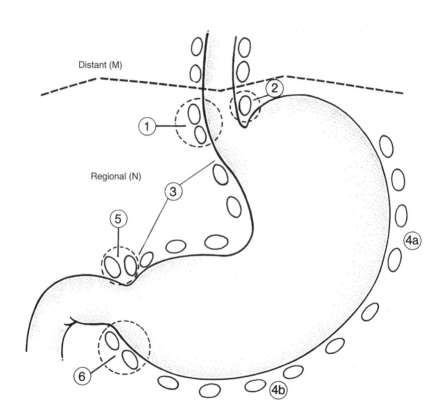

Fig. 117

Note

The numerical order corresponds to the proposals of the Japanese Gastric Cancer Society (1998) Japanese Classification of Gastric Carcinoma, 2nd English edition. Gastric Cancer 1:10–24.

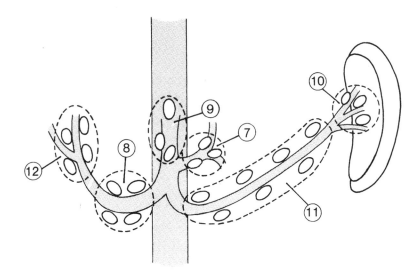

Fig. 118. Regional lymph nodes of the stomach

TNM Clinical Classification

T—Primary Tumour

TX   Primary tumour cannot be assessed
T0   No evidence of primary tumour
Tis   Carcinoma in situ: intraepithelial tumour without invasion of the lamina propria

T1   Tumour invades lamina propria or submucosa (Fig. 119)
T2   Tumour invades muscularis propria or subserosa
         T2a   Tumour invades muscularis propria (Fig. 119)
         T2b   Tumour invades subserosa (Figs. 119–121)

Note
See p. 96.

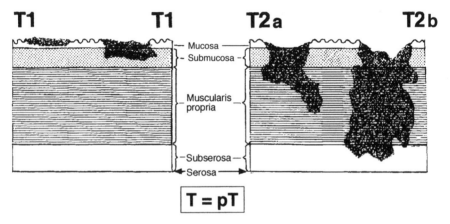

Fig. 119

T2b

pT2b

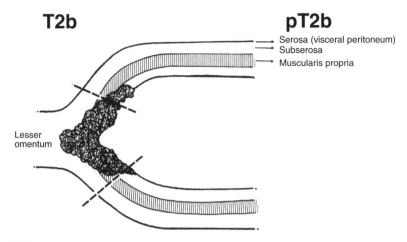

→ Serosa (visceral peritoneum)
→ Subserosa
→ Muscularis propria

Lesser omentum

Fig. 120

T2b

pT2b

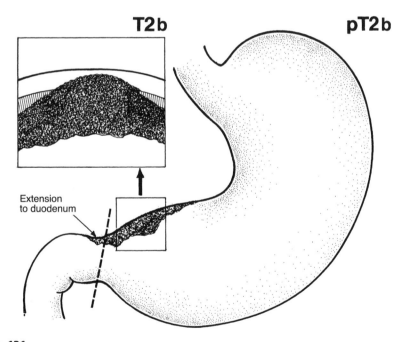

Extension to duodenum

Fig. 121

T3   Tumour penetrates serosa (visceral peritoneum) without invasion of adjacent structures[1,2,3] (Fig. 122)

T4   Tumour invades adjacent structures[1,2,3] (Fig. 122)

Note

[1] A tumour may penetrate muscularis propria with extension into the gastrocolic or gastrohepatic ligaments or the greater and lesser omentum without perforation of the visceral peritoneum covering these structures. In this case, the tumour is classified as T2b. If there is perforation of the visceral peritoneum covering the gastric ligaments or omenta, the tumour is classified as T3 (Fig. 123).

[2] The adjacent structures of the stomach are the spleen, transverse colon, liver, diaphragm, pancreas, abdominal wall, adrenal gland, kidney, small intestine, and retroperitoneum.

[3] Intramural extension to the duodenum or oesophagus is classified by the depth of greatest invasion in any of these sites including stomach (Figs. 121, 124).

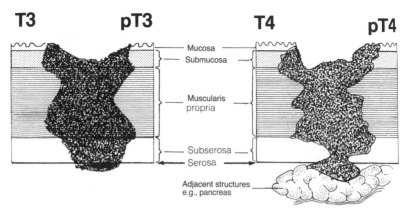

Fig. 122

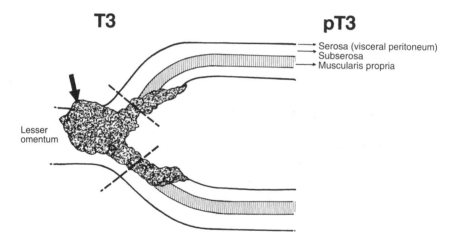

Fig. 123

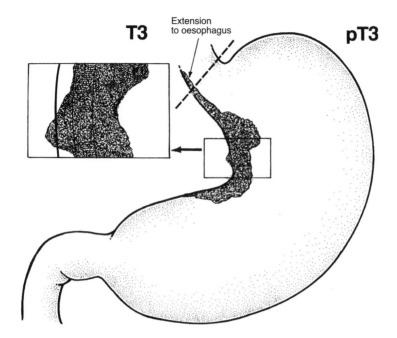

Fig. 124

N—Regional Lymph Nodes

NX   Regional lymph nodes cannot be assessed
N0   No regional lymph node metastasis
N1   Metastasis in 1 to 6 regional lymph nodes (Fig. 125)
N2   Metastasis in 7 to 15 regional lymph nodes (Fig. 126)
N3   Metastasis in more than 15 regional lymph nodes (Fig. 127)

N1

pN1

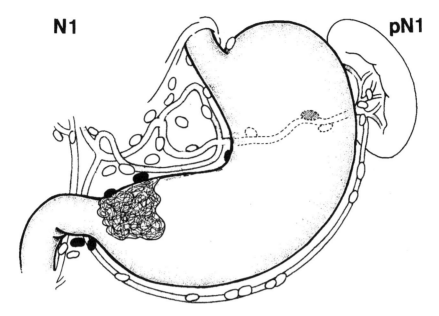

Fig. 125

N2

pN2

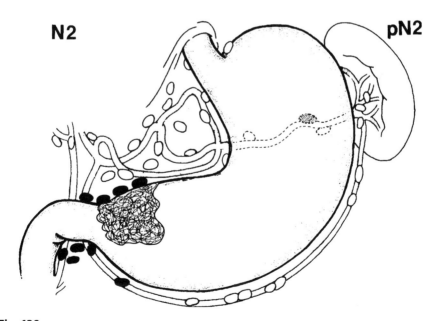

Fig. 126

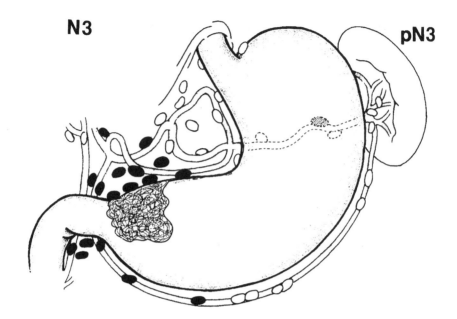

N3

pN3

Fig. 127

M—Distant Metastasis

MX   Distant metastasis cannot be assessed
M0   No distant metastasis
M1   Distant metastasis (Fig. 128)

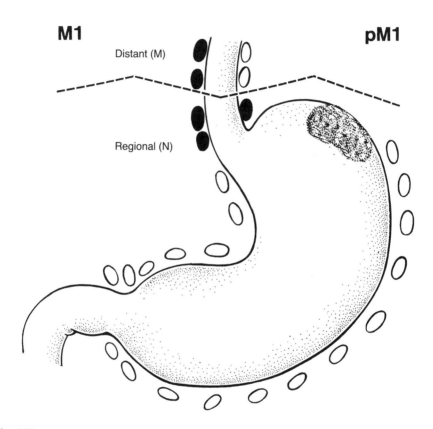

Fig. 128

pTNM Pathological Classification

The pT, pN, and pM categories correspond to the T, N, and M categories.

pN0 Histological examination of a regional lymphadenectomy specimen will ordinarily include 15 or more lymph nodes. If the examined lymph nodes are negative, but the number ordinarily resected is not met, classify as pN0.

Summary

Stomach	
T1	Lamina propria, submucosa
T2	Muscularis propria, subserosa
T2a	Muscularis propria
T2b	Subserosa
T3	Penetrates serosa
T4	Adjacent structures
N1	1 to 6 nodes
N2	7 to 15 nodes
N3	>15 nodes

Small Intestine (ICD-O C17)

Rules for Classification

The classification applies only to carcinomas. There should be histological confirmation of the disease.

Anatomical Subsites (Fig. 129)

1. Duodenum (C17.0)
2. Jejunum (C17.1)
3. Ileum (C17.2) (excludes ileocecal valve C18.0)

Note
This classification does not apply to carcinomas of the ampulla of Vater (see p. 154 ff).

Fig. 129

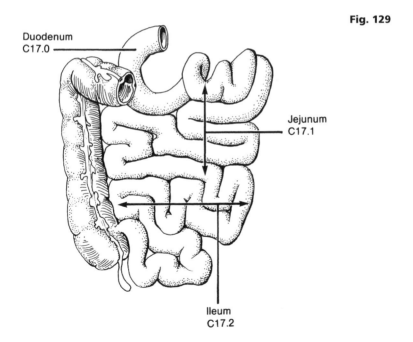

Duodenum
C17.0

Jejunum
C17.1

Ileum
C17.2

Regional Lymph Nodes

The regional lymph nodes for the duodenum are the pancreaticoduodenal, pyloric, hepatic (pericholedochal, cystic, hilar), and superior mesenteric nodes.

The regional lymph nodes for the ileum and jejunum are the mesenteric nodes, including the superior mesenteric nodes, and, for the terminal ileum only, the ileocolic nodes including the posterior cecal nodes.

TN Clinical Classification

T—Primary Tumour

TX   Primary tumour cannot be assessed
T0   No evidence of primary tumour
Tis Carcinoma in situ

T1   Tumour invades lamina propria or submucosa (Fig. 130)
T2   Tumour invades muscularis propria (Fig. 131)
T3   Tumour invades through muscularis propria into subserosa or into non-peritonealized perimuscular tissue (mesentery or retroperitoneum*) with extension 2.0 cm or less (Figs. 132, 134)
T4   Tumour perforates visceral peritoneum or directly invades other organs or structures (includes other loops of small intestine, mesentery, or retroperitoneum more than 2.0 cm and abdominal wall by way of serosa; for duodenum only, invasion of pancreas) (Figs. 133–136)

Note

* The non-peritonealized perimuscular tissue is, for jejunum and ileum, part of the mesentery and, for duodenum in areas where serosa is lacking, part of the retroperitoneum (Fig. 134).

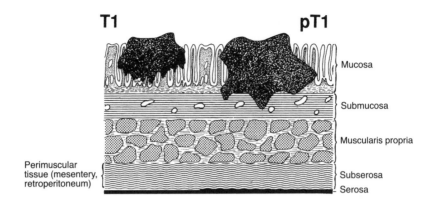

Fig. 130

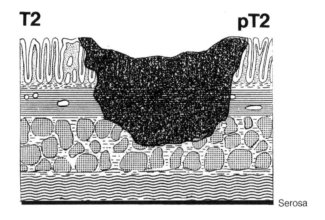

Fig. 131

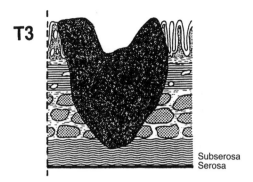

Fig. 132

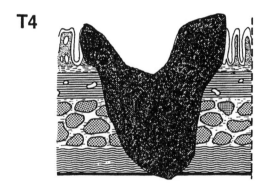

Fig. 133

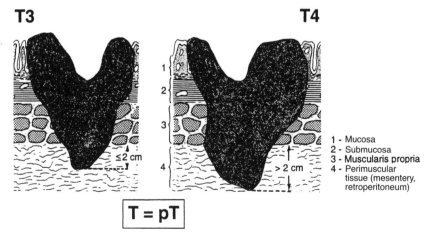

1 - Mucosa
2 - Submucosa
3 - **Muscularis propria**
4 - Perimuscular
tissue (mesentery,
retroperitoneum)

Fig. 134

pT4   Fig. 135

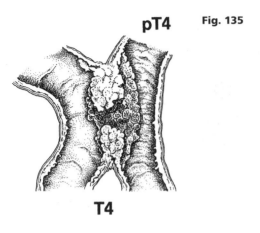

T4

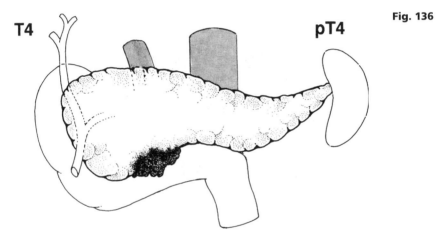

T4   pT4   Fig. 136

N—Regional Lymph Nodes

NX   Regional lymph nodes cannot be assessed
N0   No regional lymph node metastasis
N1   Regional lymph node metastasis

pTN Pathological Classification

The pT and pN categories correspond to the T and N categories.

pN0 Histological examination of a regional lymphadenectomy specimen will ordi-narily include 6 or more lymph nodes. If the examined lymph nodes are negative, but the number ordinarily resected is not met, classify as pN0.

Summary

Small Intestine	
T1	Lamina propria, submucosa
T2	Muscularis propria
T3	Subserosa, non-peritonealized perimuscular tissues (mesentery, retroperitoneum) ≤2 cm
T4	Visceral peritoneum, other organs/structures (including mesentery, retroperitoneum >2 cm)
N1	Regional

Colon and Rectum (ICD-O C18-C20)

Rules for Classification

The classification applies only to carcinomas. There should be histological confirmation of the disease.

Anatomical Subsites

Colon (Fig. 137)
1. Appendix (18.1)
2. Caecum (C18.0)
3. Ascending colon (C18.2)
4. Hepatic flexure (C18.3)
5. Transverse colon (C18.4)
6. Splenic flexure (C18.5)
7. Descending colon (C18.6)
8. Sigmoid colon (C18.7)

Rectosigmoid junction (C19) (Fig. 138)

Rectum (C20) (Fig. 138)

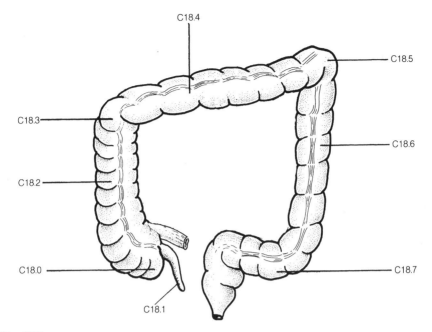

Fig. 137

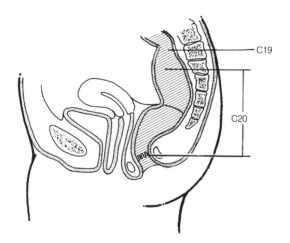

Fig. 138

Regional Lymph Nodes

For each anatomical subsite the following are the regional lymph nodes:

Appendix (Fig. 139)
    ileocolic lymph nodes

Caecum (Fig. 140)
    ileocolic, right colic lymph nodes

Ascending colon (Fig. 141)
    ileocolic, right colic, middle colic lymph nodes

Hepatic flexure (Fig. 142)
    right colic, middle colic lymph nodes

Transverse colon (Fig. 143)
    right colic, middle colic, left colic, inferior mesenteric lymph nodes

Splenic flexure (Fig. 144)
    middle colic, left colic, inferior mesenteric lymph nodes

Descending colon (Fig. 145)
    left colic, inferior mesenteric lymph nodes

Sigmoid colon (Fig. 146)
    left colic, inferior mesenteric, sigmoid, superior rectal (haemorrhoidal),
    rectosigmoid lymph nodes

Rectum (Fig. 147)
    Superior, middle, and inferior rectal (haemorrhoidal), inferior mesenteric,
    internal iliac, mesorectal (paraproctal), lateral sacral, presacral, sacral
    promotory (Gerota) lymph nodes

Metastasis in nodes other than those listed above is classified as distant metastasis
except if the primary tumour directly invades other segments of colon and rectum,
or the small intestine.

Fig. 139

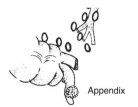

Appendix

Fig. 140

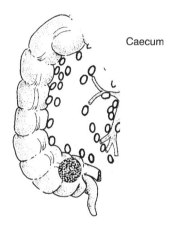

Caecum

Fig. 141

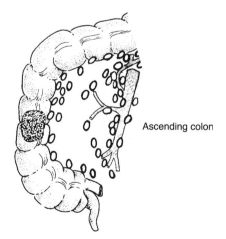

Ascending colon

Hepatic flexure   **Fig. 142**

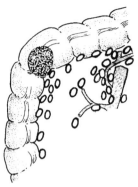

Transverse colon   **Fig. 143**

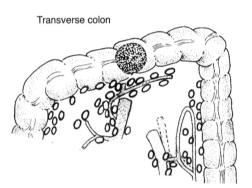

Splenic flexure **Fig. 144**

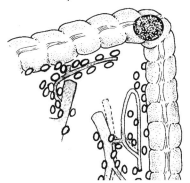

Descending colon **Fig. 145**

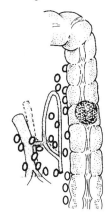

Sigmoid colon   **Fig. 146**

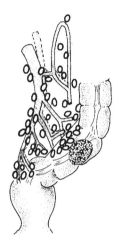

Rectum   **Fig. 147**

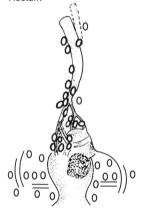

TN Clinical Classification

T—Primary Tumour

TX   Primary tumour cannot be assessed
T0   No evidence of primary tumour
Tis   Carcinoma in situ: intraepithelial or invasion of lamina propria[1]

T1   Tumour invades submucosa (Fig. 148)
T2   Tumour invades muscularis propria (Fig. 149)

Note
[1] Tis includes cancer cells confined within the glandular basement membrane (intraepithelial) or lamina propria (intramucosal) with no extension through muscularis mucosae into submucosa.

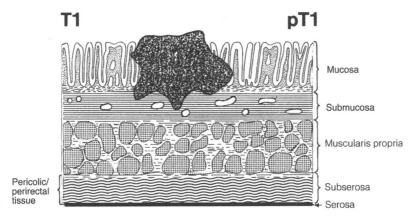

Fig. 148

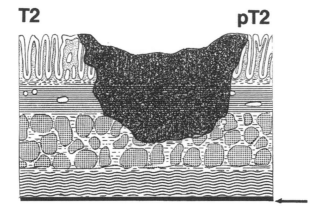

Fig. 149

T3 Tumour invades through muscularis propria into subserosa or into non-peritonealized pericolic or perirectal tissues (Fig. 150)

T4 Tumour directly invades other organs or structures[2,3] and/or perforates visceral peritoneum (Figs. 151, 152)

Note

[2] Direct invasion in T4 includes invasion of other segments of the colorectum by way of the serosa, e.g. invasion of sigmoid colon by a carcinoma of the caecum.

[3] Tumour that is adherent to other organs or structures macroscopically is classified T4; however, if no tumour is present in the adhesion microscopically, the classification would be pT3.

T3   pT3   **Fig. 150**

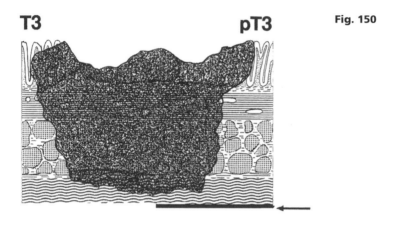

T4   pT4   **Fig. 151**

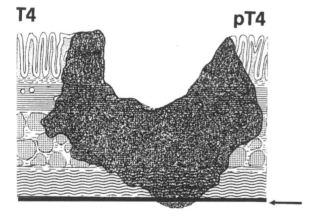

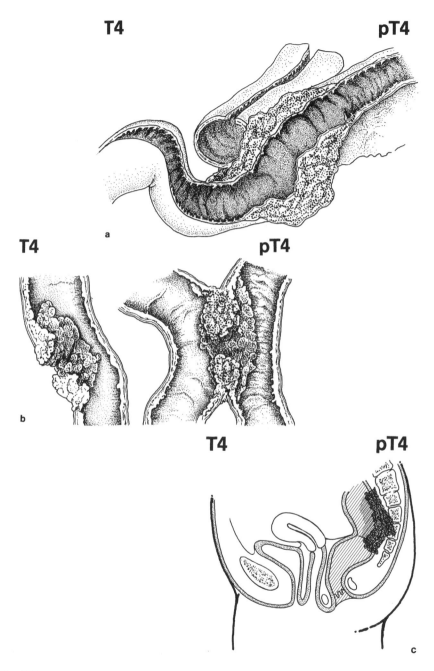

T4   **pT4**

T4   **pT4**

T4   **pT4**

Fig. 152a–c

N—Regional Lymph Nodes

NX Regional lymph nodes cannot be assessed
N0 No regional lymph node metastasis
N1 Metastasis in 1 to 3 regional lymph nodes (Fig. 153)
N2 Metastasis in 4 or more regional lymph nodes (Figs. 154–156)

Note

A tumour nodule in pericolic/perirectal adipose tissue of a primary carcinoma without histological evidence of a residual lymph node in the nodule is classified in the pN category as regional lymph node metastasis if the nodule has the form and smooth contour of a lymph node. If the nodule has an irregular contour, it should be classified in the pT category and also coded as V1 (microscopic venous invasion) or V2, if it was grossly evident, because there is a strong likelihood that it represents venous invasion.

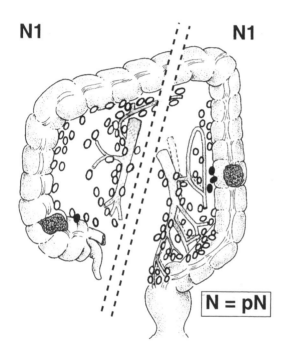

N1   **N1**   **Fig. 153**

N = pN

N2 **N2**

Fig. 154

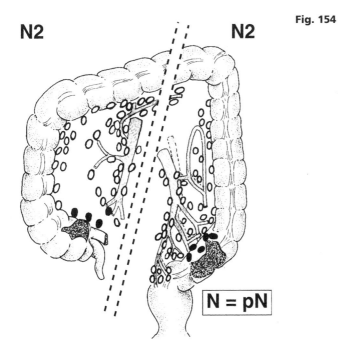

N = pN

N2 **N2**

Fig. 155

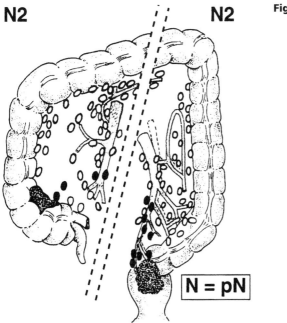

N = pN

N2   **pN2**   **Fig. 156.** Apical node involvement does not
                                                     alter the classification

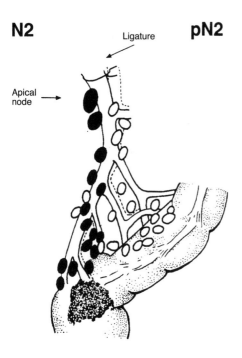

pTN Pathological Classification

The pT and pN categories correspond to the T and N categories.

pN0 Histological examination of a regional lymphadenectomy specimen will ordinarily include 12 or more lymph nodes. If the examined lymph nodes are negative, but the number ordinarily resected is not met, classify as pN0.

Summary

Colon and Rectum	
T1	Submucosa
T2	Muscularis propria
T3	Subserosa, non-peritonealized pericolic/perirectal tissues
T4	Other organs or structures/visceral peritoneum
N1	≤ 3 regional
N2	>3 regional

Anal Canal (ICD-O C21.1, 2)

The anal canal (Fig. 157) extends from rectum to perianal skin (to the junction with hair-bearing skin). It is lined by the mucous membrane overlying the internal sphincter, including the transitional epithelium and dentate line. Tumours of anal margin (ICD-O C44.5) are classified with skin tumours (p. 211 ff.).

Rules for Classification

The classification applies only to carcinomas. There should be histological confirmation of the disease.

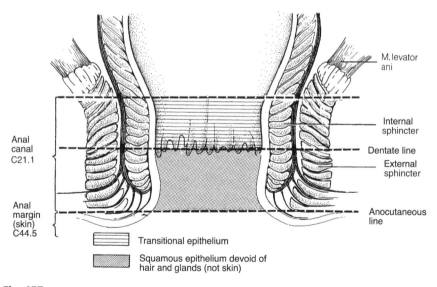

Fig. 157

124

Regional Lymph Nodes (Fig. 158)

The regional lymph nodes are the perirectal (1), the internal iliac (2), and the inguinal (3) lymph nodes.

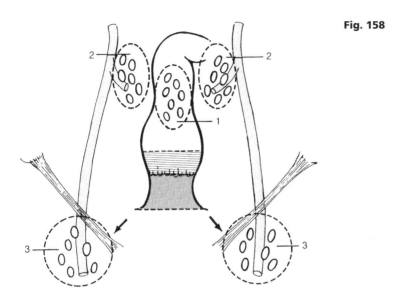

Fig. 158

TN Clinical Classification

T—Primary Tumour

TX   Primary tumour cannot be assessed
T0   No evidence of primary tumour
Tis   Carcinoma in situ

T1   Tumour 2.0 cm or less in greatest dimension (Fig. 159)
T2   Tumour more than 2.0 cm but not more than 5.0 cm in greatest dimension (Fig. 160)
T3   Tumour more than 5 cm in greatest dimension (Fig. 161)

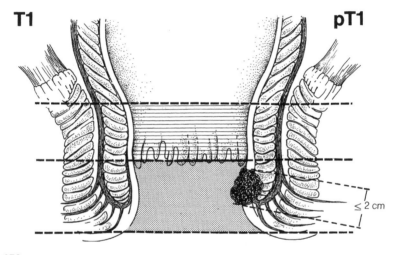

Fig. 159

T2 T2

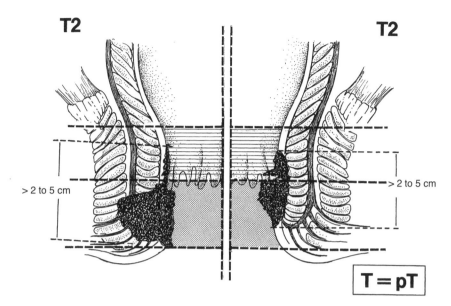

> 2 to 5 cm

> 2 to 5 cm

T = pT

Fig. 160

T3 pT3

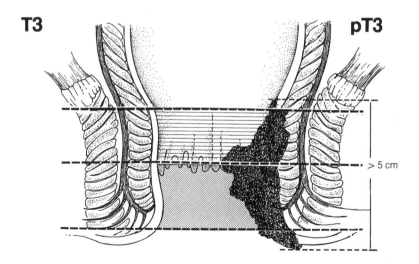

> 5 cm

Fig. 161

T4   Tumour of any size invades adjacent organ(s), e.g., vagina, urethra, bladder
      (Fig. 162)

Note
Direct invasion of the rectal wall, perirectal skin, subcutaneous tissue or the sphincter muscle(s) alone is
not classified as T4.

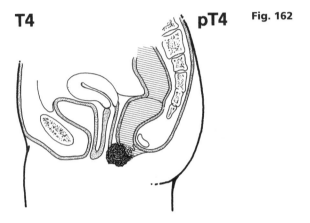

Fig. 162

N—Regional Lymph Nodes

NX   Regional lymph nodes cannot be assessed
N0   No regional lymph node metastasis
N1   Metastasis in perirectal lymph node(s) (Fig. 163)

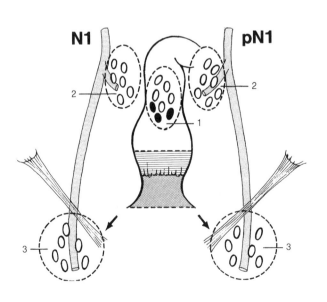

Fig. 163

N2   Metastasis in unilateral internal iliac and/or inguinal lymph node(s) (Figs. 164, 165)

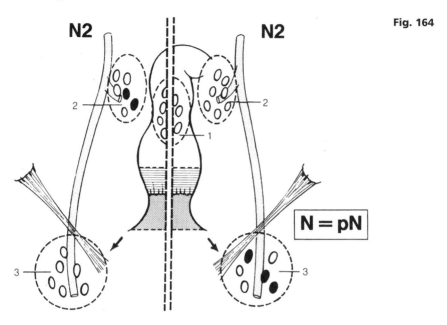

Fig. 164

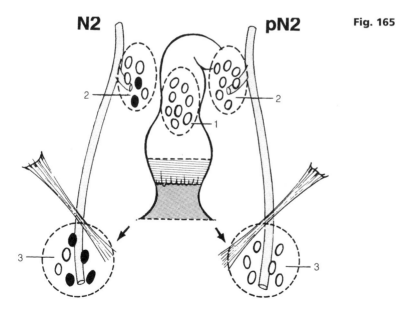

Fig. 165

N3   Metastasis in perirectal and inguinal lymph nodes and/or bilateral internal
       iliac and/or inguinal lymph nodes (Figs. 166–168)

Fig. 166

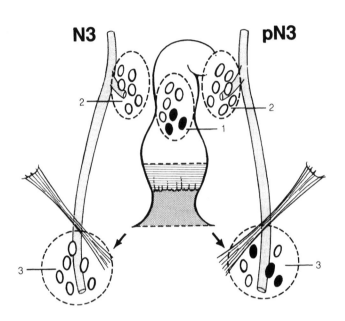

Fig. 167

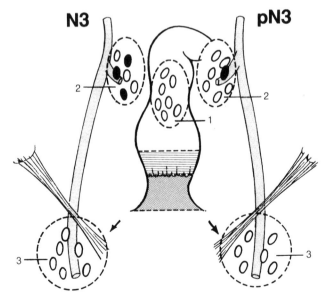

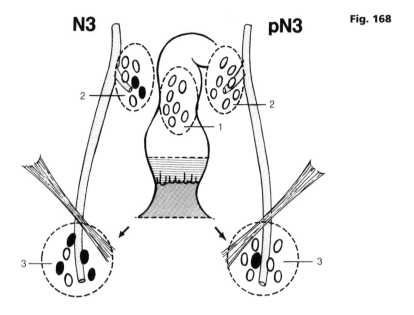

N3   pN3   Fig. 168

pTN Pathological Classification

The pT and pN categories correspond to the T and N categories.

pN0 Histological examination of a regional perirectal-pelvic lymphadenectomy specimen will ordinarily include 12 or more lymph nodes; histological examination of an inguinal lymphadenectomy specimen will ordinarily include 6 or more lymph nodes. If the examined lymph nodes are negative, but the number ordinarily resected is not met, classify as pN0.

Summary

Anal Canal	
T1	≤2 cm
T2	>2 to 5 cm
T3	>5 cm
T4	Adjacent organ(s)
N1	Perirectal
N2	Unilateral internal iliac/inguinal
N3	Perirectal and inguinal, bilateral internal iliac/inguinal

Liver (ICD-O C22)

Rules for Classification

The classification is intended primarily for hepatocellular carcinoma. It may also be used for cholangio- (intrahepatic bile duct) carcinoma of the liver. There should be histological confirmation of the disease and division of cases by histological type.

Anatomical Subsites (Fig. 169)

1. Liver (C22.0)
2. Intrahepatic bile duct (C22.1)

Regional Lymph Nodes (Fig. 169)

The regional lymph nodes are the hilar, hepatic (along the proper hepatic artery), periportal (along the portal vein) nodes and those along the abdominal inferior vena cava above the renal vein (except the inferior phrenic nodes).

Fig. 169

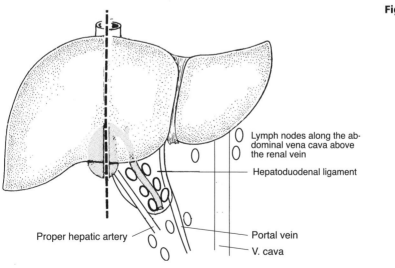

Lymph nodes along the abdominal vena cava above the renal vein

Hepatoduodenal ligament

Proper hepatic artery

Portal vein

V. cava

133

TN Clinical Classification

T—Primary Tumour

TX   Primary tumour cannot be assessed
T0   No evidence of primary tumour

T1   Solitary tumour without vascular invasion (Fig. 170)

Fig. 170

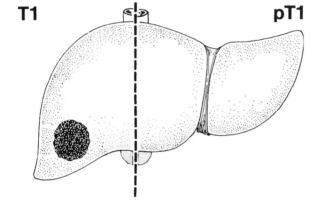

T2 Solitary tumour with vascular invasion; *or* multiple tumours none more than 5 cm in greatest dimension (Figs. 171, 172)

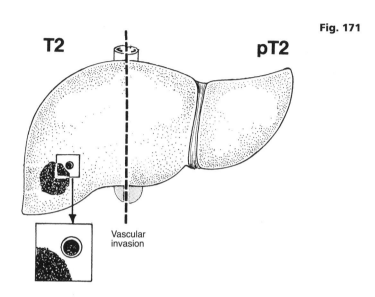

Fig. 171

Vascular
invasion

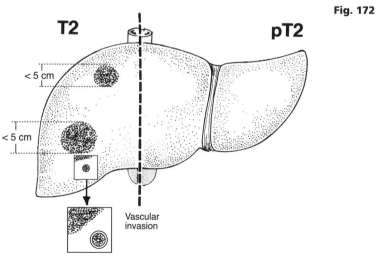

Fig. 172

Vascular
invasion

T3   Multiple tumours more than 5.0 cm or tumour involving a major branch of
      the portal or hepatic vein(s) (Figs. 173–175)

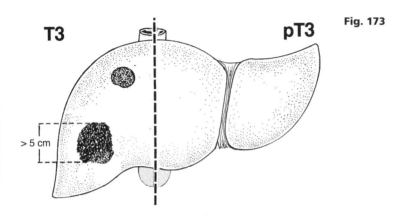

Fig. 173

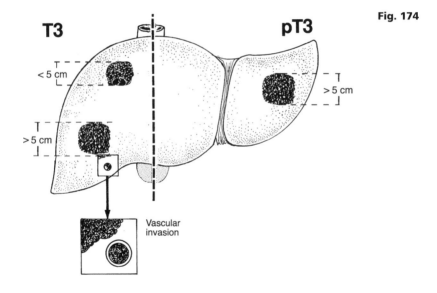

Fig. 174

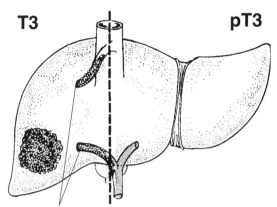

T3   pT3   **Fig. 175**

Major branch of the portal or hepatic vein (s)

T4   Tumour(s) with direct invasion of other organs other than gallbladder *or* with
      perforation of visceral peritoneum (Fig. 176)

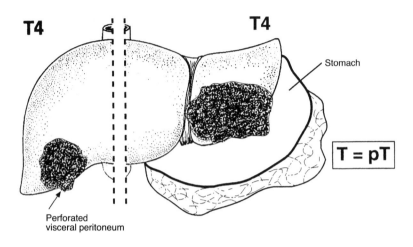

Fig. 176

N—Regional Lymph Nodes

NX   Regional lymph nodes cannot be assessed
N0   No regional lymph node metastasis
N1   Regional lymph node metastasis

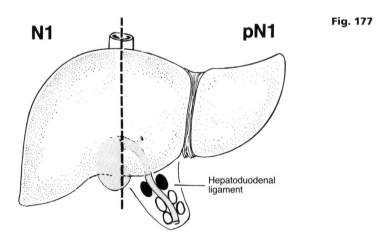

Fig. 177

pTN Pathological Classification

The pT and pN categories correspond to the T and N categories.

pN0 Histological examination of a regional lymphadenectomy specimen will ordinarily include 3 or more lymph nodes. If the examined lymph nodes are negative, but the number ordinarily resected is not met, classify as pN0.

Summary

Liver	
T1	Solitary without vascular invasion
T2	Solitary with vascular invasion
	Multiple ≤5 cm
T3	Multiple >5 cm
	Invades major branch of portal or hepatic vein(s)
T4	Invades adjacent organs other than gallbladder
	Perforates visceral peritoneum
N1	Regional

Gallbladder (ICD-O C23.9)

Rules for Classification

The classification applies only to carcinomas. There should be histological confirmation of the disease.

Regional Lymph Nodes (Fig. 178)

The regional lymph nodes are the cystic duct node and the pericholedochal, hilar, peripancreatic (head only), periduodenal, periportal, coeliac, and superior mesenteric nodes.

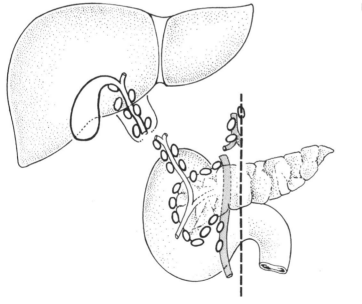

Fig. 178

TN Clinical Classification

T—Primary Tumour

TX   Primary tumour cannot be assessed
T0   No evidence of primary tumour
Tis   Carcinoma in situ

T1   Tumour invades lamina propria or muscle layer (Fig. 179)
T1a   Tumour invades lamina propria
T1b   Tumour invades muscle layer

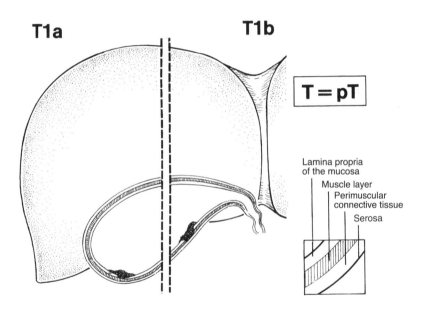

Fig. 179

T2   Tumour invades perimuscular connective tissue, no extension beyond serosa
     or into liver (Fig. 180)

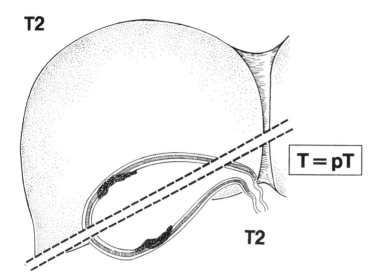

T2

Fig. 180

T = pT

T2

T3   Tumour perforates serosa (visceral peritoneum) and/or directly invades the
      liver and/or one other adjacent organ or structure, e.g., stomach, duodenum,
      colon, pancreas, omentum, extrahepatic bile ducts (Figs. 181, 182)

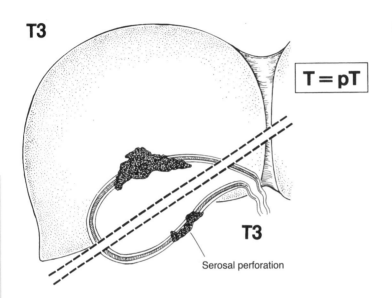

T3   **Fig. 181**

T = pT

T3

Serosal perforation

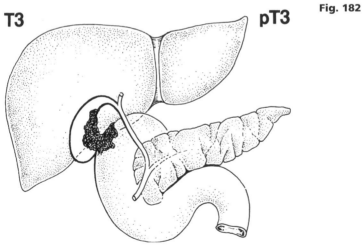

T3   **pT3**   **Fig. 182**

T4   Tumour invades main portal vein or hepatic artery, or invades two or more
       extrahepatic organs or structures (Figs. 183, 184)

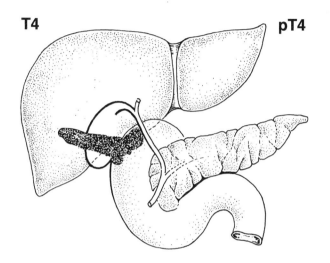

Fig. 183. Invasion of duodenum and extrahepatic bile duct

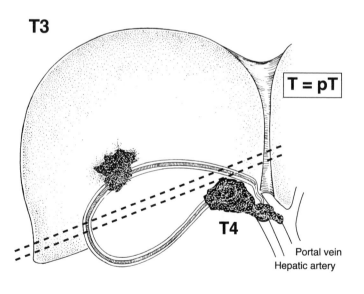

Fig. 184

Portal vein
Hepatic artery

N—Regional Lymph Nodes (Figs. 185, 186)

NX   Regional lymph nodes cannot be assessed
N0   No regional lymph node metastasis
N1   Regional lymph node metastasis

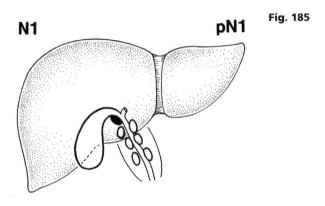

N1   **pN1**   **Fig. 185**

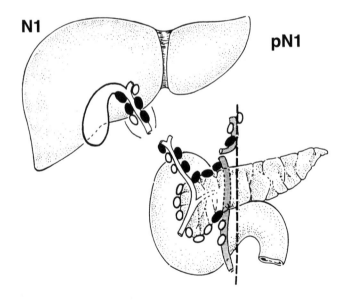

Fig. 186

N1

pN1

pTN Pathological Classification

The pT and pN categories correspond to the T and N categories.

pN0 Histological examination of a regional lymphadenectomy specimen will ordinarily include 3 or more lymph nodes. If the examined lymph nodes are negative, but the number ordinarily resected is not met, classify as pN0.

Summary

Gallbladder	
T1	Gallbladder wall
T1a	Lamina propria
T1b	Muscle
T2	Perimuscular connective tissue
T3	Serosa, one organ and/or liver
T4	Portal vein, hepatic artery, or two or more extrahepatic organs
N1	Regional

Extrahepatic Bile Ducts (ICD-O C24.0)

Rules for Classification

The classification applies to carcinomas of extrahepatic bile ducts and those of choledochal cysts. There should be histological confirmation of the disease.

Anatomic subsites (Fig. 187)

1. Right hepatic duct
2. Left hepatic duct
3. Common hepatic duct
4. Common bile duct
5. Cystic duct

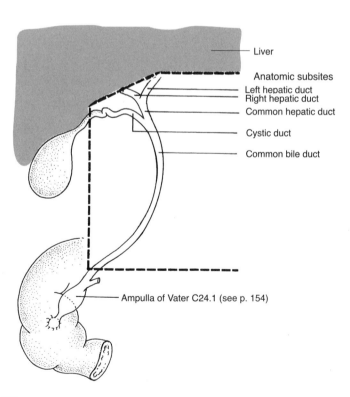

Liver

Anatomic subsites
Left hepatic duct
Right hepatic duct
Common hepatic duct

Cystic duct

Common bile duct

Ampulla of Vater C24.1 (see p. 154)

Fig. 187

Regional Lymph Nodes (Fig. 187, p. 129)

The regional lymph nodes are the cystic duct, pericholedochal, hilar, peripancreatic (head only), periduodenal, periportal, coeliac, and superior mesenteric nodes.

TN Clinical Classification

T—Primary Tumour

TX   Primary tumour cannot be assessed
T0   No evidence of primary tumour
Tis   Carcinoma in situ

T1   Tumour confined to the wall of the bile duct[1] (Fig. 188)
T2   Tumour invades beyond the wall of the bile duct (Fig. 189)

Note
[1] The "wall of the bile duct" includes epithelium, subepithelial connective tissue and the fibromuscular layer.

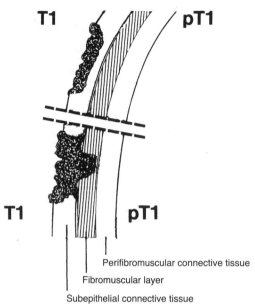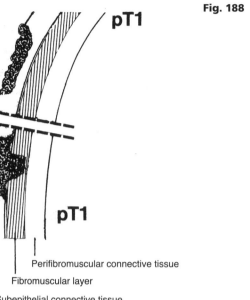

Fig. 188

Perifibromuscular connective tissue

Fibromuscular layer

Subepithelial connective tissue

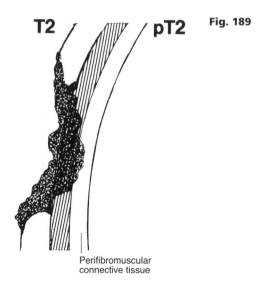

Fig. 189

Perifibromuscular
connective tissue

T3   Tumour invades the liver, gallbladder, pancreas, and/or unilateral tributaries of the portal vein (right or left) or hepatic artery (right or left) (Fig. 190)

T4   Tumour invades any of the following: main portal vein or its tributaries bilaterally, common hepatic artery, or other adjacent structures, e.g., colon, stomach, duodenum, abdominal wall (Fig. 191)

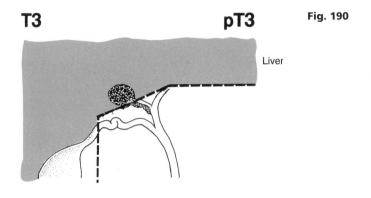

T3   **pT3**   **Fig. 190**

Liver

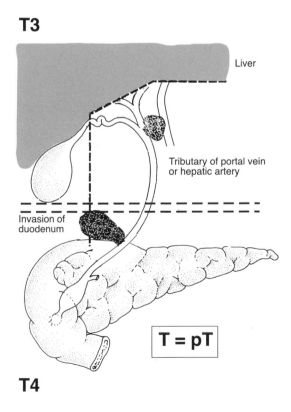

T3

Liver

Tributary of portal vein
or hepatic artery

Invasion of
duodenum

$T = pT$

T4

Fig. 191

N—Regional Lymph Nodes

NX   Regional lymph nodes cannot be assessed
N0   No regional lymph node metastasis
N1   Regional lymph node metastasis (Figs. 185, 186, p. 146)

pTN Pathological Classification

The pT and pN categories correspond to the T and N categories.

pN0 Histological examination of a regional lymphadenectomy specimen will ordinarily include 3 or more lymph nodes. If the examined lymph nodes are negative, but the number ordinarily resected is not met, classify as pN0.

Summary

Extrahepatic Bile Ducts	
T1	Ductal wall
T2	Beyond ductal wall
T3	Liver, gallbladder, pancreas, or unilateral vessels
T4	Other adjacent organs, or main or bilateral vessels
N1	Regional

Ampulla of Vater (ICD-O C24.1) (Fig. 192)

Rules for Classification

The classification applies only to carcinomas. There should be histological confirmation of the disease.

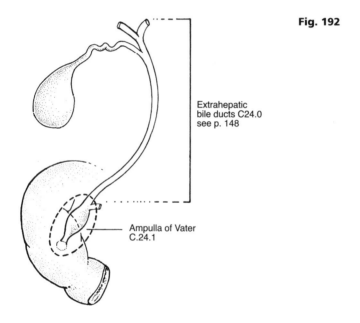

Fig. 192

Extrahepatic
bile ducts C24.0
see p. 148

Ampulla of Vater
C.24.1

Regional Lymph Nodes (Fig. 193a, b)

The regional lymph nodes are:

Superior   Superior to head (1) and body (2) of pancreas
Inferior   Inferior to head (3) and body (4) of pancreas

Anterior   Anterior pancreaticoduodenal (5), pyloric (6, not shown in Fig. 193a, b) and proximal mesenteric (7)

Posterior   Posterior pancreaticoduodenal (8), common bile duct (9), and proximal mesenteric (7)

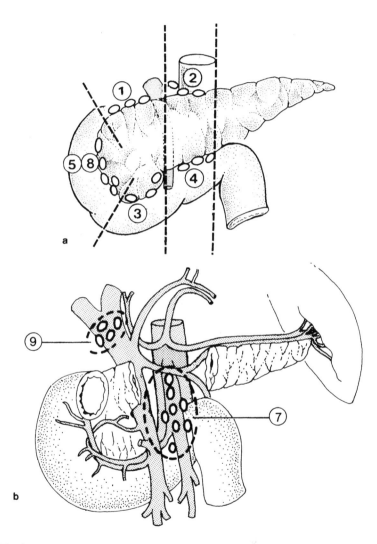

Fig. 193a, b

Note

The splenic lymph nodes and those of the tail of the pancreas are not regional; metastases to these lymph nodes are coded M1.

TNM Clinical Classification

T—Primary Tumour

TX   Primary tumour cannot be assessed
T0   No evidence of primary tumour
Tis   Carcinoma in situ

T1   Tumour limited to ampulla of Vater or sphincter of Oddi (Fig. 194)
T2   Tumour invades duodenal wall (Fig. 195)

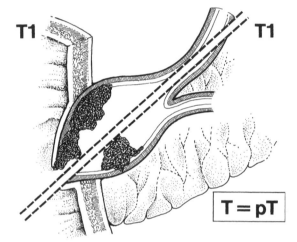

Fig. 194

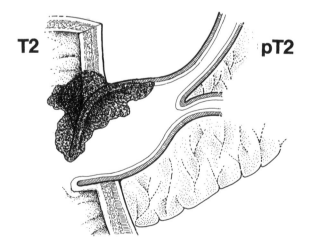

Fig. 195

T3   Tumour invades pancreas (Fig. 196)

T4   Tumour invades peripancreatic soft tissues, or other adjacent organs or
structures (Fig. 197)

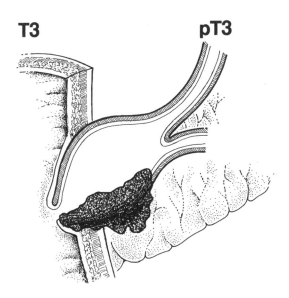

Fig. 196

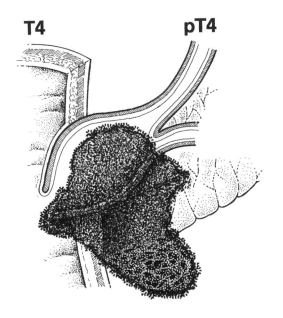

Fig. 197

N—Regional Lymph Nodes

NX   Regional lymph nodes cannot be assessed
N0   No regional lymph node metastasis
N1   Regional lymph node metastasis (Figs. 198, 199a, b)

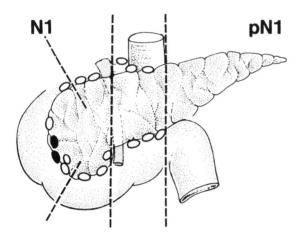

Fig. 198

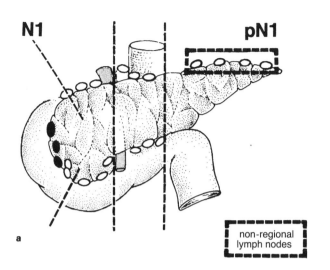

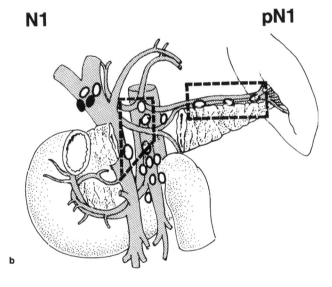

M—Distant Metastasis

MX   Distant metastasis cannot be assessed
M0   No distant metastasis
M1   Distant metastasis (Fig. 200) (includes metastasis in splenic lymph nodes
      and/or those at the tail of the pancreas)

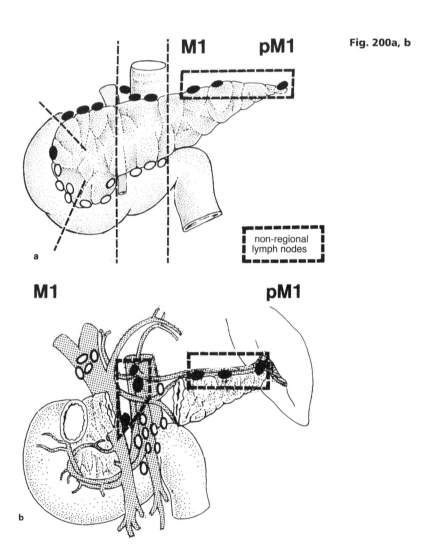

Fig. 200a, b

pTNM Pathological Classification

The pT, pN and pM categories correspond to the T, N and M categories.

pN0 Histological examination of a regional lymphadenectomy specimen will ordinarily include 10 or more lymph nodes. If the examined lymph nodes are negative, but the number ordinarily resected is not met, classify as pN0.

Summary

Ampulla of Vater	
T1	Ampulla or sphincter of Oddi
T2	Duodenal wall
T3	Pancreas
T4	Beyond pancreas
N1	Regional

Pancreas (ICD-O C25.0–2, 8)

Rules for Classification

The classification applies only to carcinomas of the exocrine pancreas. There should be histological or cytological confirmation of the disease.

Anatomical Subsites (Fig. 201)

1. Head of pancreas[1] (C25.0)
2. Body of pancreas[2] (C25.1)
3. Tail of pancreas[3] (C25.2)

Notes

[1] Tumours of the head of the pancreas are those arising to the right of the left border of the superior mesenteric vein. The uncinate process is considered as part of the head.

[2] Tumours of the body are those arising between the left border of the superior mesenteric vein and left border of the aorta.

[3] Tumours of the tail are those arising between the left border of the aorta and the hilum of the spleen.

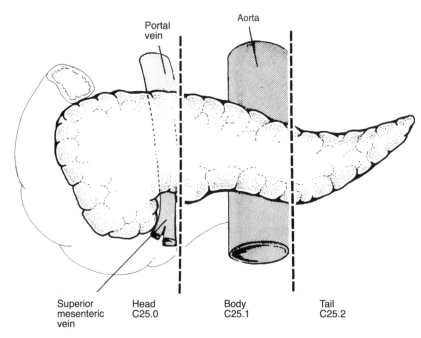

Fig. 201

Regional Lymph Nodes (Fig. 202a, b)

The regional lymph nodes are the peripancreatic nodes, which may be subdivided as follows:

Superior: Superior to head (1) and body (2)
Inferior: Inferior to head (3) and body (4)
Anterior: Anterior pancreaticoduodenal (5), pyloric (for tumours of head only) (6, not shown in Fig. 202), and proximal mesenteric (7)
Posterior: Posterior pancreaticoduodenal (8), common bile duct (9), and proximal mesenteric (7)
Splenic: Hilum of spleen (10) and tail of pancreas (11) (for tumours of body and tail only)
Coeliac: for tumours of head only (12)

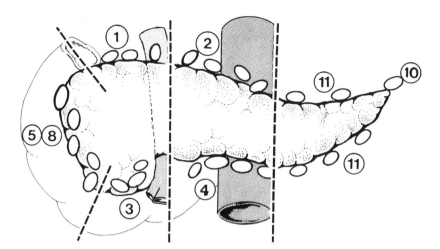

Fig. 202a

Fig. 202b

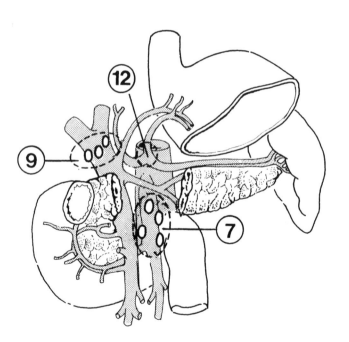

TN Clinical Classification

T—Primary Tumour

TX   Primary tumour cannot be assessed
T0   No evidence of primary tumour
Tis   Carcinoma in situ

T1   Tumour limited to the pancreas, 2.0 cm or less in greatest dimension (Fig. 203)
T2   Tumour limited to the pancreas, more than 2.0 cm in greatest dimension (Fig. 203)

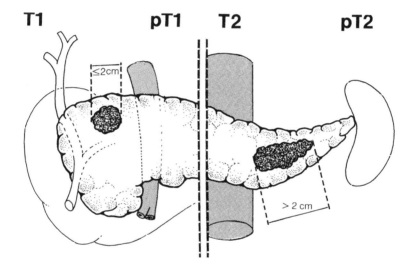

Fig. 203

T3   Tumour extends beyond pancreas, but without involvement of coeliac axis or
      superior mesenteric artery (Fig. 204)
T4   Tumour involves coeliac axis or superior mesenteric artery (Fig. 205)

T3   **pT3**

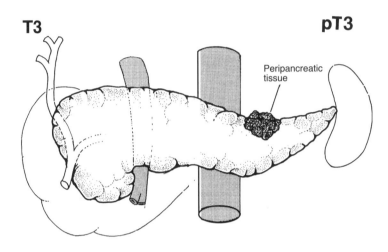

Peripancreatic
tissue

Fig. 204

T4   **pT4**   **Fig. 205**

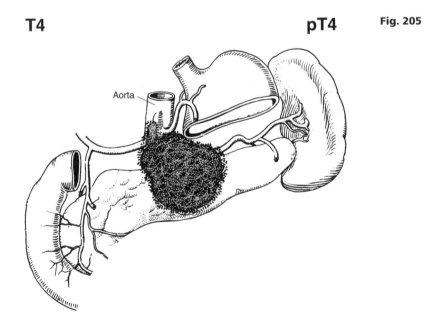

Aorta

N—Regional Lymph Nodes

NX   Regional lymph nodes cannot be assessed
N0   No regional lymph node metastasis
N1   Regional lymph node metastasis (Figs. 206, 207)

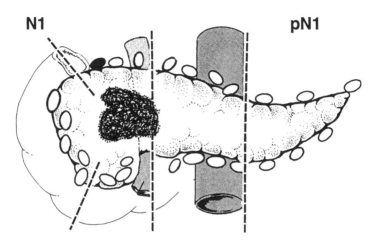

Fig. 206

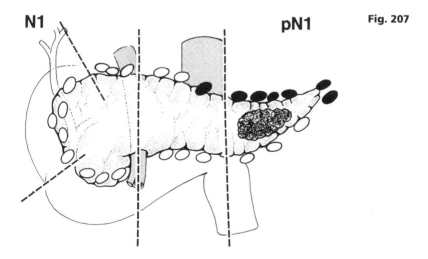

Fig. 207

pTN Pathological Classification

The pT and pN categories correspond to the T and N categories.

pN0 Histological examination of a regional lymphadenectomy specimen will ordinarily include 10 or more lymph nodes. If the examined lymph nodes are negative, but the number ordinarily resected is not met, classify as pN0.

Summary

Pancreas	
T1	Limited to pancreas ≤2 cm
T2	Limited to pancreas >2 cm
T3	Beyond pancreas
T4	Coeliac axis or superior mesenteric artery
N1	Regional

Lung and Pleural Tumours

Introductory Notes

The classifications apply to carcinomas of the lung and malignant mesothelioma of pleura.

Regional Lymph Nodes (Figs. 208, 209)

The regional lymph nodes for lung tumors are the intrathoracic, scalene, and supraclavicular nodes, for pleural mesothelioma in addition the internal mammary nodes.

The intrathoracic nodes include:
a) *Mediastinal nodes* (Figs. 208, 209)
    (1) highest (superior) mediastinal
    (2) paratracheal (upper tracheal)
    (3) pretracheal
    (3a) anterior mediastinal
    (3b) retrotracheal (posterior mediastinal)
    (4) tracheobronchial (lower paratracheal) (including azygos nodes)
    (5) subaortic (aortic window)
    (6) para-aortic (ascending aorta or phrenic)
    (7) subcarinal
    (8) paraoesophageal (below carina)
    (9) pulmonary ligament
b) *Peribronchial and hilar nodes* (Figs. 208, 209)
    (10) hilar (main bronchus)
    (11) interlobar
    (12) lobar
    (13) segmental
    (14) subsegmental

Direct extension of the primary tumour into lymph nodes is classified as lymph node metastasis.

TNM Atlas: Illustrated Guide to the TNM Classification of Malignant Tumours, Fifth Edition,
edited by Christian Wittekind, Frederick L. Greene, Robert Hutter, Martin Klimpfinger, and Leslie H. Sobin
Copyright © 2005 UICC

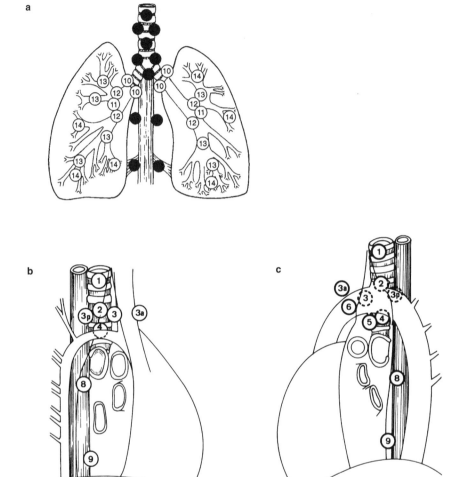

Fig. 208a-c. Lymph node map of Naruke. [Modified from Naruke T, Suemasu K, Ishikawa S (1978) Lymph node mapping and curability at various levels of metastasis in resected lung cancer. J Thorac Cardiovasc Surg 76: 832–839]

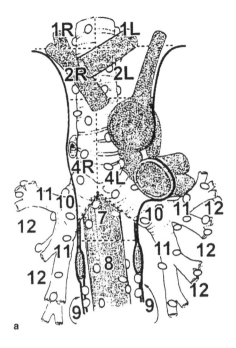

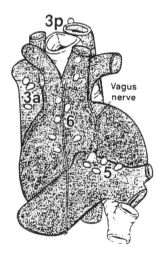

N2 Lymph Nodes

Superior mediastinal lymph nodes

1. Highest mediastinal

2. Upper paratracheal

3. Pre- and retrotracheal

4. Lower paratracheal (including azygos nodes)

Aortic lymph nodes

5. Subaortic (A-P windows)

6. Paraaortic (ascending aorta or phrenic)

Inferior mediastinal lymph nodes

7. Subcarinal

8. Paraoesophageal (below carina)

9. Pulmonary ligament

N1 Lymph nodes

10. Hilar

11. Interlobar

12. Lobar

13. Segmental

14. Subsegmental

Fig. 209a, b. Regional lymph nodes for lung cancer. Used with the permission of the American Joint Committee on Cancer (AJCC), Chicago, Illinois. The original source for the material is the AJCC Cancer Staging Manual, 6th edition (2002) Greene FL, Page DL, Fleming ID, Fritz AG, Balch CM, Haller DG Morrow M (eds) Springer, New York

Lung (ICD-O C34)

Rules for Classification

The classification applies only to carcinomas. There should be histological confirmation of the disease and division of cases by histological type.

Anatomical Subsites (Fig. 210)

1. Main bronchus (C34.0)
2. Upper lobe (C34.1)
3. Middle lobe (C34.2)
4. Lower lobe (C34.3)

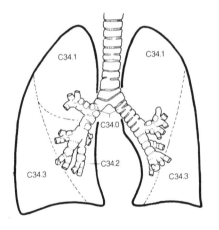

Fig. 210

Regional Lymph Nodes

The regional lymph nodes are the intrathoracic, scalene, and supraclavicular nodes (see pp. 171–173).

TNM Clinical Classification

T—Primary Tumour

TX Primary tumour cannot be assessed, *or* tumour proven by the presence of malignant cells in
    sputum or bronchial washings but not visualized by imaging or bronchoscopy
T0 No evidence of primary tumour
Tis Carcinoma in situ

T1 Tumour 3.0 cm or less in greatest dimension, surrounded by lung or
    visceral pleura, without bronchoscopic evidence of invasion more proximal
    than the lobar bronchus (i.e., not in the main bronchus)[1] (Fig. 211)
T2 Tumour with *any* of the following features of size or extent:
    - More than 3.0 cm in greatest dimension (Fig. 212)
    - Involves main bronchus, 2.0 cm or more distal to the carina
    - Invades visceral pleura
    - Associated with atelectasis or obstructive pneumonitis that extends to
      the hilar region but does not involve the entire lung

T3 Tumour of any size that directly invades any of the following: chest wall
    (including superior sulcus tumours), diaphragm, mediastinal pleura,
    parietal pericardium; *or* tumour in the main bronchus less than 2.0 cm
    distal to the carina[1] but without involvement of the carina; *or* associated
    atelectasis or obstructive pneumonitis of the entire lung (Fig. 213)
T4 Tumour of any size that invades any of the following: mediastinum, heart,
    great vessels, trachea, oesophagus, vertebral body, carina; separate tumour
    nodule(s) in the same lobe; tumour with malignant pleural effusion[2]
    (Figs. 214–222)

Note

[1] The uncommon superficial spreading tumour of any size with its invasive component limited to the
bronchial wall, which may extend proximal to the main bronchus, is also classified as T1.

[2] Most pleural effusions with lung cancer are due to tumour. In a few patients, however, multiple
cytopathological examinations of pleural fluid are negative for tumour, and the fluid is non-bloody and
is not an exudate. Where these elements and clinical judgment dictate that the effusion is not related to
the tumour, the effusion should be excluded as a staging element and the patient should be classified as
T1, T2, or T3.

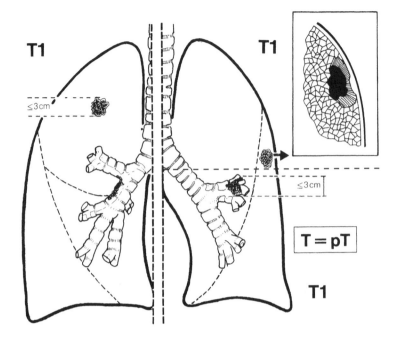

Fig. 211

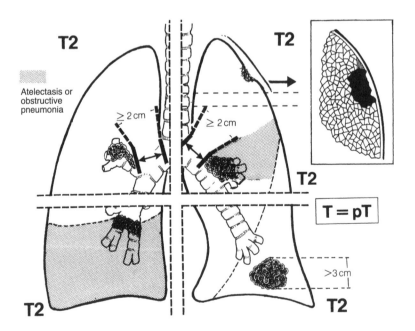

Fig. 212

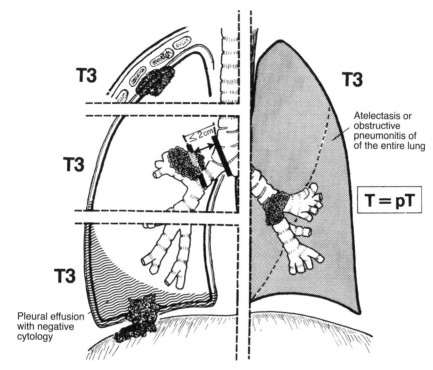

Fig. 213

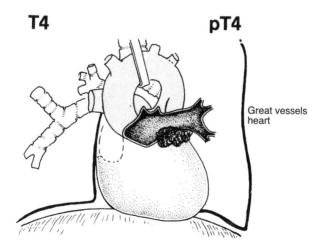

Fig. 214

T4   pT4

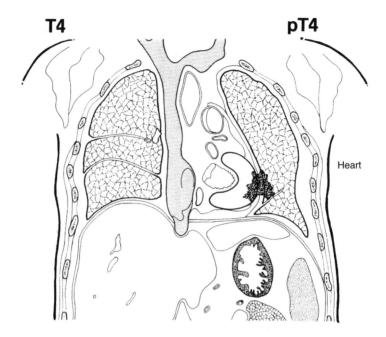

Heart

Fig. 215

T4   pT4

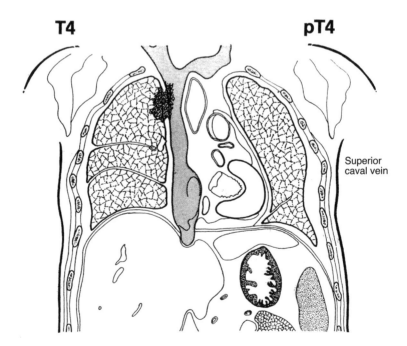

Superior
caval vein

Fig. 216

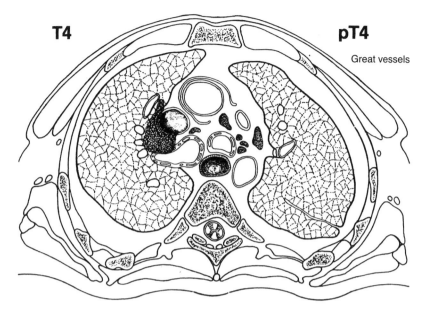

T4 pT4

Great vessels

Fig. 217

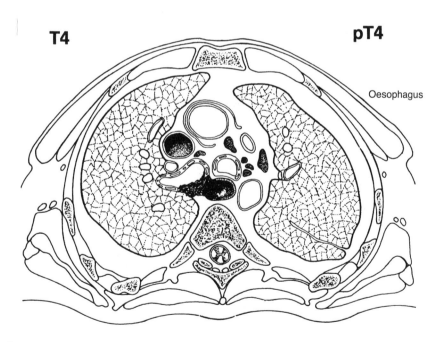

T4 pT4

Oesophagus

Fig. 218

T4   **pT4**

Vertebral
body

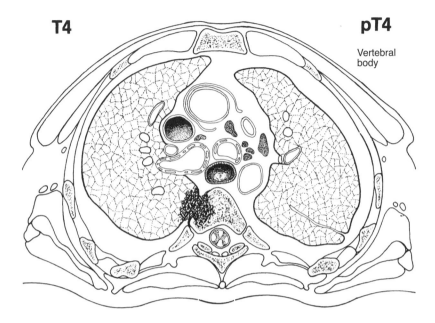

Fig. 219

T4   **M1**

T = pT

M = pM

Primary
tumour

Primary
tumour

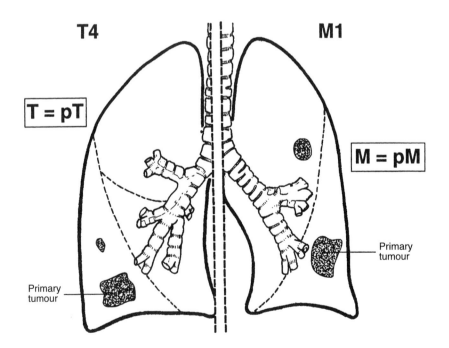

Fig. 220

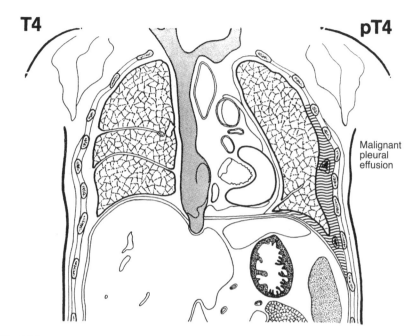

T4   **pT4**

Malignant
pleural
effusion

Fig. 221

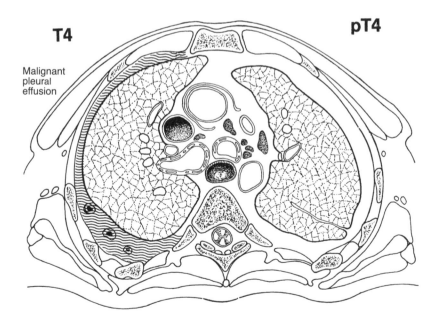

T4   **pT4**

Malignant
pleural
effusion

Fig. 222

N—Regional Lymph Nodes

NX   Regional lymph nodes cannot be assessed
N0   No regional lymph node metastasis
N1   Metastasis in ipsilateral peribronchial and/or ipsilateral hilar lymph nodes
       and intrapulmonary nodes, including involvement by direct extension
       (Fig. 223)

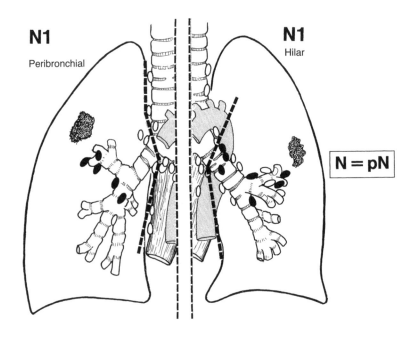

Fig. 223

N2   Metastasis in ipsilateral mediastinal and/or subcarinal lymph
      node(s) (Fig. 224)

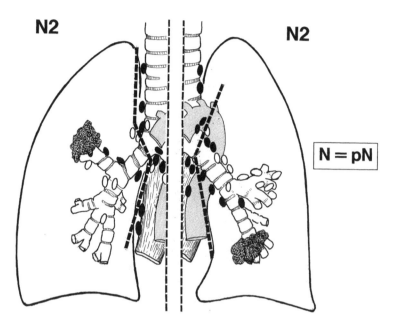

Fig. 224

N3   Metastasis in contralateral mediastinal, contralateral hilar, ipsilateral or
            contralateral scalene, or supraclavicular lymph node(s) (Fig. 225)

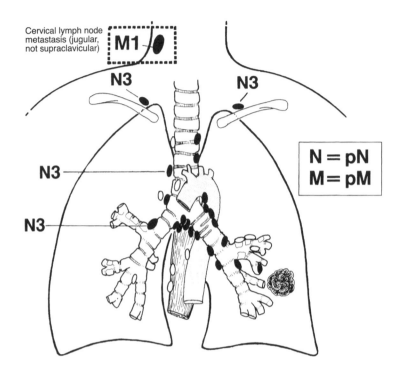

Fig. 225

M—Distant Metastasis

MX   Distant metastasis cannot be assessed
M0   No distant metastasis
M1   Distant metastasis, includes separate tumour nodule(s) in a different lobe
        (ipsilateral or contralateral) (Figs. 220, 225)

pTNM Pathological Classification

The pT, pN, and pM categories correspond to the T, N, and M categories.

pN0 Histological examination of hilar and mediastinal lymphadenectomy speci-
men(s) will ordinarily include 6 or more lymph nodes. If the examined lymph nodes
are negative, but the number ordinarily resected is not met, classify as pN0. The
number of lymph nodes should be recorded in the pathology report.

Summary

Lung	
TX	Positive cytology only
T1	≤3 cm
T2	>3 cm, main bronchus ≤2 cm from carina, invades visceral pleura, partial atelectasis
T3	Chest wall, diaphragm, pericardium, mediastinal pleura, main bronchus <2 cm from carina, total atelectasis
T4	Mediastinum, heart, great vessels, carina, trachea, oesophagus, vertebra; separate nodules in same lobe, malignant pleural effusion
N1	Ipsilateral peribronchial, ipsilateral hilar
N2	Ipsilateral mediastinal, subcarinal
N3	Contralateral mediastinal or hilar, scalene or supraclavicular
M1	Includes separate nodule in different lobe

Pleural Mesothelioma (ICD-O C38.4)

Rules for Classification

The classification applies only to malignant mesothelioma of the pleura. There should be histological confirmation of the disease.

Regional Lymph Nodes

The regional lymph nodes are the intrathoracic, internal mammary, scalene, and supraclavicular nodes (see pp. 155–157).

TN Clinical Classification

T—Primary Tumour

TX   Primary tumour cannot be assessed
T0   No evidence of primary tumour

T1   Tumour involves ipsilateral parietal pleura with or without focal involvement of visceral pleura (Fig. 226)
        T1a Tumour involves ipsilateral parietal (mediastinal, diaphragmatic) pleura. No involvement of visceral pleura (Fig. 226)
        T1b Tumour involves ipsilateral parietal (mediastinal, diaphragmatic) pleura, with focal involvement of visceral pleura (Fig. 226)

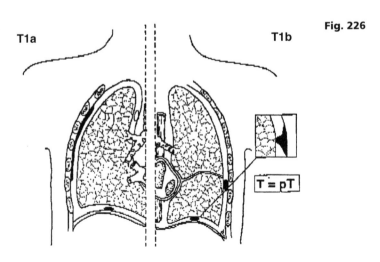

Fig. 226

T1a   T1b   T = pT

T2   Tumour involves any of the ipsilateral pleural surfaces, with at least one of
        the following:
        – confluent visceral pleural tumour including the fissure (Fig. 227)
        – invasion of diaphragmatic muscle (Fig. 228)
        – invasion of lung parenchyma (Fig. 229)

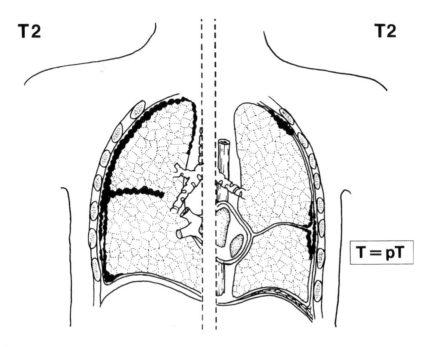

Fig. 227

T2

T2

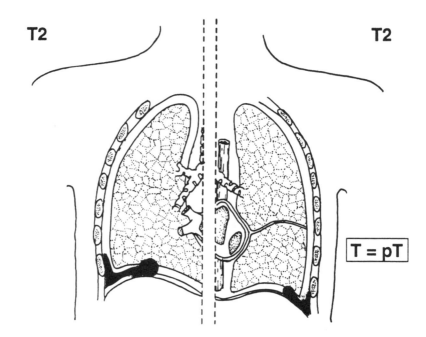

T = pT

Fig. 228

T2

T2

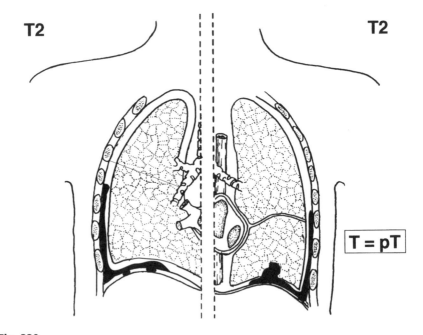

T = pT

Fig. 229

T3* Tumour involves any of the ipsilateral pleural surfaces, with at least one of the following:
  – invasion of endothoracic fascia (Fig. 230)
  – invasion of mediastinal fat (Fig. 231)
  – solitary focus of tumour invading soft tissue of the chest wall (Fig. 230)
  – non-transmural involvement of pericardium (Fig. 231)

Note
See p. 191

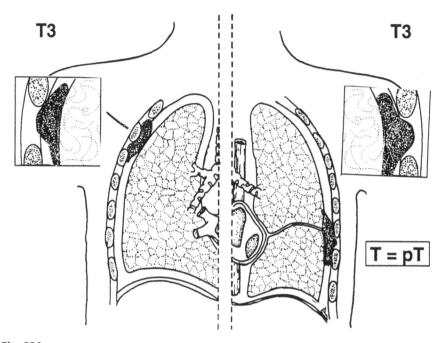

Fig. 230

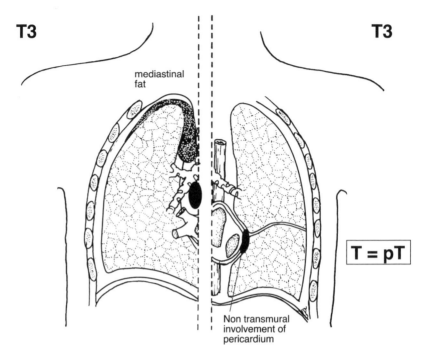

Fig. 231

T4**   Tumour involves any of the ipsilateral pleural surfaces, with at least one of
        the following:
        – diffuse or multifocal invasion of soft tissues of the chest wall (Fig. 232)
        – any involvement of rib (Fig. 232)
        – invasion through the diaphragm to the peritoneum (Fig. 233, 235)
        – invasion of any mediastinal organ(s) (Fig. 234)
        – direct extension to contralateral pleura (Fig. 235)
        – invasion into the spine (Fig. 234)
        – extension to the internal surface of the pericardium (Fig. 234)
        – pericardial effusion with positive cytology
        – invasion of the myocardium (Fig. 235)
        – invasion of the brachial plexus (Fig. 233)

Notes
* T3 describes locally advanced, but potentially resectable tumour
** T4 describes locally advanced, technically unresectable tumour

T4   pT4

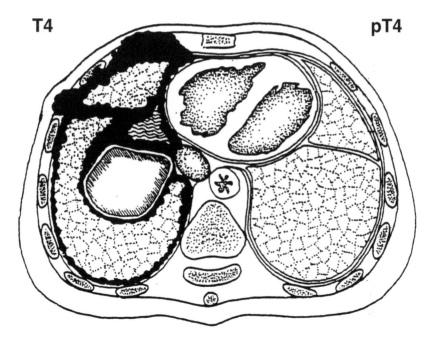

Fig. 232

T4   pT4   Fig. 233

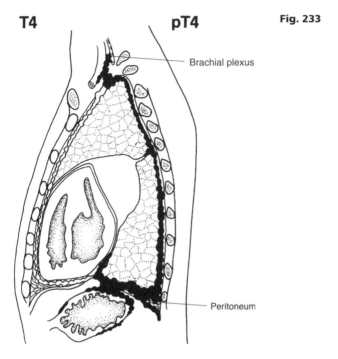

Brachial plexus

Peritoneum

T4   pT4   Fig. 234

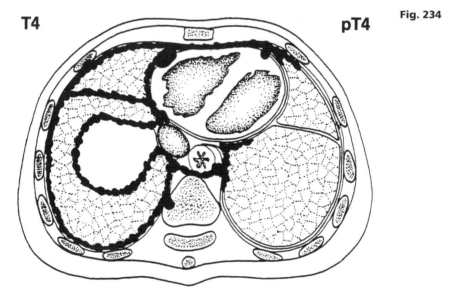

Direct extension to contralateral pleura

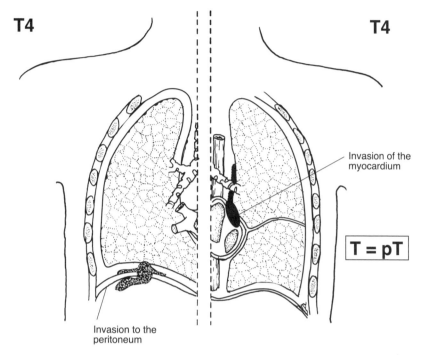

T4

T4

Invasion of the
myocardium

T = pT

Invasion to the
peritoneum

Fig. 235

N—Regional Lymph Nodes

NX   Regional lymph nodes cannot be assessed
N0   No regional lymph node metastasis

N1   Metastasis in ipsilateral peribronchial and/or ipsilateral hilar lymph nodes,
       including involvement by direct extension (Fig. 223, p. 182)
N2   Metastasis in subcarinal lymph node(s) and/or ipsilateral internal
       mammary or mediastinal lymph node(s)
N3   Metastasis in contralateral mediastinal, internal mammary, or hilar
       node(s) and/or ipsilateral or contralateral supraclavicular or scalene
       lymph node(s).

pTN Pathological Classification

The pT and pN categories correspond to the T and N categories.

Summary

Pleural Mesothelioma	
T1	Ipsilateral parietal pleura
T1a	No visceral pleura
T1b	Visceral pleura
T2	Ipsilateral lung, diaphragm, confluent involvement of visceral pleura
T3	Endothoracic fascia, mediastinal fat, focal chest wall, non-transmural pericardium
T4	Contralateral pleura, peritoneum, rib, extensive chest wall or mediastinal invasion, myocardium, brachial plexus, spine, transmural pericardium, malignant pericardial effusion
N1	Ipsilateral bronchopulmonary, hilar
N2	Subcarinal, ipsilateral mediastinal, internal mammary
N3	Contralateral mediastinal, internal mammary, hilar; ipsi/contralateral supraclavicular, scalene

Tumours of Bone and Soft Tissues

Introductory Notes

The following sites are included:

- Bone
- Soft tissue

Regional Lymph Nodes

The regional lymph nodes are those appropriate to the site of the primary tumour. Regional lymph node metastasis is rare.

The definitions of the N categories for all tumours of bone and soft tissues are:

N—Regional Lymph Nodes

NX   Regional lymph nodes cannot be assessed
N0   No regional lymph node metastasis
N1   Regional lymph node metastasis

TNM Atlas: Illustrated Guide to the TNM Classification of Malignant Tumours, Fifth Edition,
edited by Christian Wittekind, Frederick L. Greene, Robert Hutter, Martin Klimpfinger, and Leslie H. Sobin
Copyright © 2005 UICC

Bone (ICD-O C40, 41)

Rules for Classification

The classification applies to all primary malignant bone tumours except malignant lymphomas, multiple myeloma, surface/juxtacortical osteosarcoma, and juxtacortical chondrosarcoma. There should be histological confirmation of the disease and division of cases by histological type and grade.

T Clinical Classification

T—Primary Tumour

TX   Primary tumour cannot be assessed
T0   No evidence of primary tumour

T1   Tumour 8 cm or less in greatest dimension (Fig. 236)
T2   Tumour more than 8 cm in greatest dimension (Fig. 237)
T3   Discontinuous tumours in the primary bone site (Fig. 238)

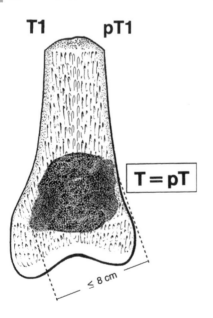

Fig. 236

T1   pT1

T = pT

≤ 8 cm

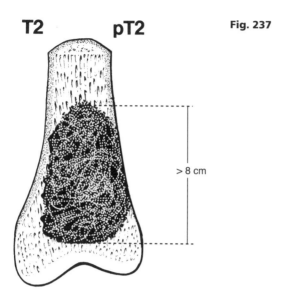

T2　　**pT2**　　　Fig. 237

> 8 cm

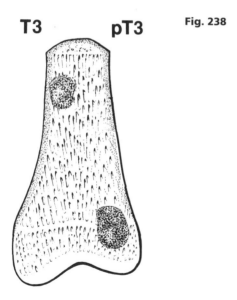

T3　　**pT3**　　Fig. 238

pT Pathological Classification

The pT categories correspond to the T categories.

Summary

Bone	
T1	≤8 cm
T2	>8 cm
T3	Discontinuous tumours in primary site
N1	Regional
M1a	Lung
M1b	Other sites
	Low grade
	High grade

Soft Tissues (ICD-O C38.1–3, C47-49)

Rules for Classification

There should be histological confirmation of the disease and division of cases by histological type and grade.

Anatomical Sites and Subsites

1. Connective, subcutaneous, and other soft tissues (C49), peripheral nerves (C47)
2. Retroperitoneum (C48)
3. Mediastinum: anterior (38.1), posterior (C38.2), mediastinum NOS (C38.3)

Histological Types of Tumour

The following histological types of malignant tumour are included, the appropriate ICD-O morphology rubrics being indicated:

Alveolar soft part sarcoma	9581/3
Epithelioid sarcoma	8804/3
Extraskeletal chondrosarcoma	9220/3
Extraskeletal osteosarcoma	9180/3
Extraskeletal Ewing sarcoma	9260/3
Primitive neuroectodermal tumour (PNET)	9473/3
Fibrosarcoma	8810/3
Leiomyosarcoma	8890/3
Liposarcoma	8850/3
Malignant fibrous histiocytoma	8830/3
Malignant hemangiopericytoma	9150/3
Malignant mesenchymoma	8990/3
Malignant peripheral nerve sheath tumour	9540/3
Rhabdomyosarcoma	8900/3
Synovial sarcoma	9040/3
Sarcoma NOS (not otherwise specified)	8800/3

The following histological types are not included: Kaposi sarcoma, dermatofibrosarcoma (protuberans), fibromatosis (desmoid tumour), and sarcoma arising from the dura mater, brain, hollow viscera, or parenchymatous organs (with the exception of breast sarcomas). Angiosarcoma, an aggressive sarcoma, is excluded because its natural history is not consistent with classification.

T Clinical Classification

T—Primary Tumour

TX   Primary tumour cannot be assessed
T0   No evidence of primary tumour

T1   Tumour 5.0 cm or less in greatest dimension
      T1a   Superficial tumour* (Fig. 239)
      T1b   Deep tumour* (Fig. 240)
T2   Tumour more than 5.0 cm in greatest dimension
      T2a   Superficial tumour* (Fig. 239)
      T2b   Deep tumour* (Fig. 240)

Note
* Superficial tumour is located exclusively above the superficial fascia without invasion of the fascia; deep tumour is located either exclusively beneath the superficial fascia or superficial to the fascia with invasion of or through the fascia. Retroperitoneal, mediastinal, and pelvic sarcomas are classified as deep tumours.

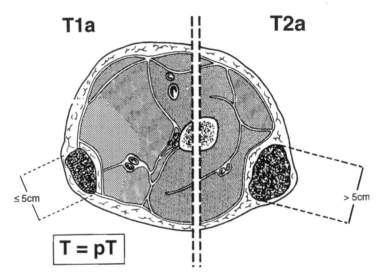

Fig. 239

T1b   pT1b

Fig. 240

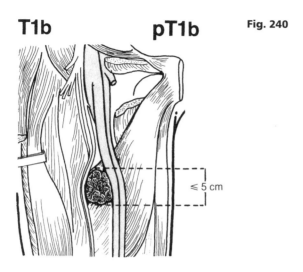

≤ 5 cm

T2b   pT2b

Fig. 241

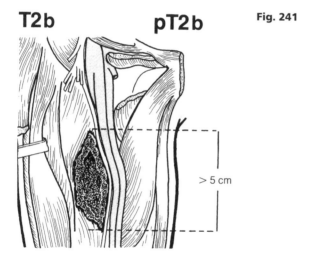

> 5 cm

pT Pathological Classification

The pT categories correspond to the T categories.

Summary

Soft Tissues	
T1	≤5 cm
T1a	Superficial
T1b	Deep
T2	>5 cm
T2a	Superficial
T2b	Deep
N1	Regional
	Low grade
	High grade

Skin Tumours

Introductory Notes

The classifications apply to carcinomas of the skin, excluding eyelid (see p. 378), vulva (see p. 248), and penis (see p. 305) and to malignant melanomas of the skin including eyelid.

Anatomical Sites

The following sites are identified by ICD-O topography rubrics:

- Lip (excluding vermilion surface) (C44.0)
- Eyelid (C44.1)
- External ear (C44.2)
- Other and unspecified parts of face (C44.3)
- Scalp and neck (C44.4)
- Trunk including anal margin and perianal skin (C44.5)
- Upper limb and shoulder (C44.6)
- Lower limb and hip (C44.7)
- Vulva (C51.0)
- Penis (C60.9)
- Scrotum (C63.2)

TNM Atlas: Illustrated Guide to the TNM Classification of Malignant Tumours, Fifth Edition,
edited by Christian Wittekind, Frederick L. Greene, Robert Hutter, Martin Klimpfinger, and Leslie H. Sobin
Copyright © 2005 UICC

Regional Lymph Nodes (Figs. 242, 243a, b)

The regional lymph nodes are those appropriate to the site of the primary tumour.

Unilateral Tumours

Head, neck:	Ipsilateral preauricular, submandibular, cervical, and supraclavicular lymph nodes
Thorax:	Ipsilateral axillary lymph nodes
Upper limb:	Ipsilateral epitrochlear and axillary lymph nodes
Abdomen, loins, and buttocks:	Ipsilateral inguinal lymph nodes
Lower limb:	Ipsilateral popliteal and inguinal lymph nodes
Anal margin and perianal skin:	Ipsilateral inguinal lymph nodes

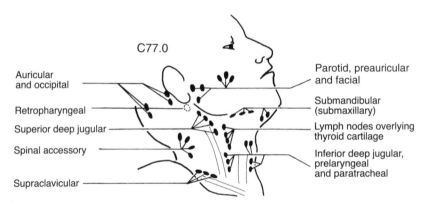

C77.0

Auricular and occipital

Retropharyngeal

Superior deep jugular

Spinal accessory

Supraclavicular

Parotid, preauricular and facial

Submandibular (submaxillary)

Lymph nodes overlying thyroid cartilage

Inferior deep jugular, prelaryngeal and paratracheal

Fig. 242

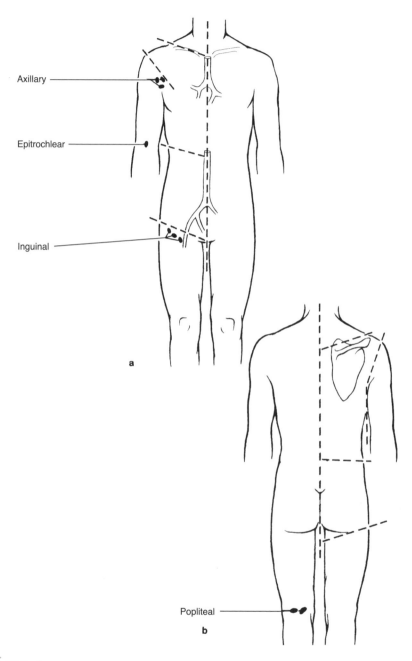

Axillary

Epitrochlear

Inguinal

a

Popliteal

b

Fig. 243a, b

Tumours in the Boundary Zones

The lymph nodes pertaining to the regions on both sides of the boundary zone are considered to be the regional lymph nodes. The following 4-cm-wide bands are considered as boundary zones (Figs. 243–248):

Between	*Along*
Right/left	Midline
Head and neck/thorax	Clavicula–acromion–upper shoulder blade edge
Thorax/upper limb	Shoulder–axilla–shoulder
Thorax/abdomen, loins, and buttocks	*Front:* middle between navel and costal arch
	Back: lower border of thoracic vertebrae (midtransverse axis)
Abdomen, loins, and buttock/lower limb	Groin–trochanter–gluteal sulcus

Any metastasis to other than the listed regional lymph nodes is considered as M1 (Figs. 244–248).

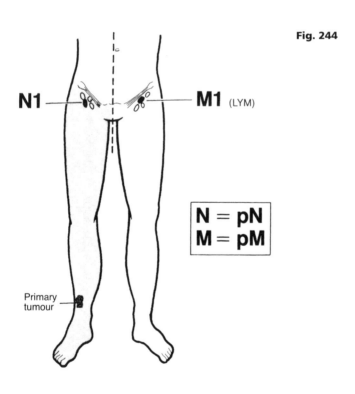

Fig. 244

N1

M1 (LYM)

$$N = pN$$
$$M = pM$$

Primary tumour

Fig. 245

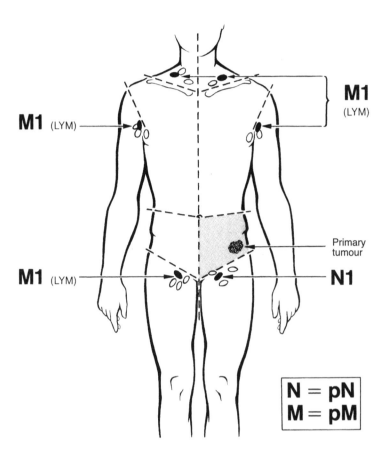

M1
(LYM)

M1 (LYM)

M1 (LYM)

Primary
tumour

N1

N = pN
M = pM

Skin Tumours

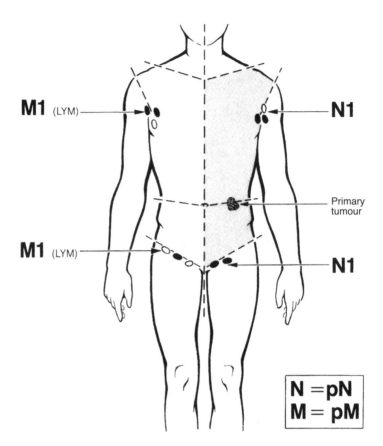

M1 (LYM)

N1

M1 (LYM)

N1

Primary tumour

N = pN
M = pM

Fig. 246

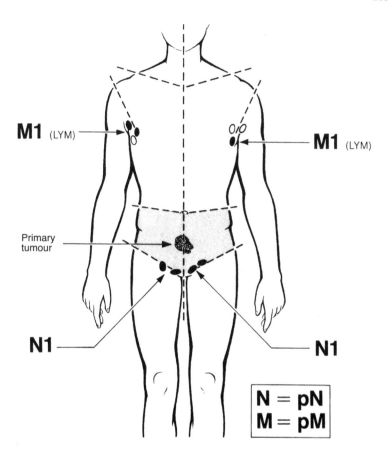

Fig. 247

Fig. 248

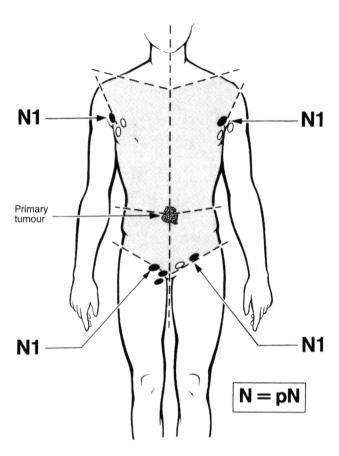

N1

N1

Primary
tumour

N1

N1

N = pN

Carcinoma of the Skin

(excluding eyelid, vulva, and penis) (ICD-O C44.0, 2–9, C63.2)

Rules for Classification

The classification applies only to carcinomas. There should be histological confirmation of the disease and division of cases by histological type.

Regional Lymph Nodes

The regional lymph nodes are those appropriate to the site of the primary tumour. (See p. 204)

TNM Clinical Classification

T—Primary Tumour

TX   Primary tumour cannot be assessed
T0   No evidence of primary tumour
Tis   Carcinoma in situ(Fig. 249)

Tis   **pTis**   Fig. 249

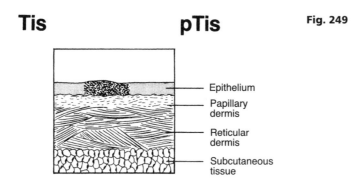

- Epithelium
- Papillary dermis
- Reticular dermis
- Subcutaneous tissue

T1   Tumour 2 cm or less in greatest dimension (Fig. 250)
T2   Tumour more than 2 cm but not more than 5 cm in greatest dimension
        (Fig. 251)
T3   Tumour more than 5 cm in greatest dimension (Fig. 252)

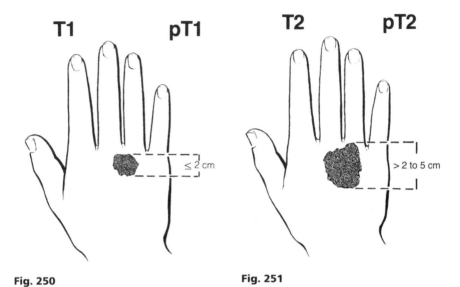

Fig. 250   **Fig. 251**

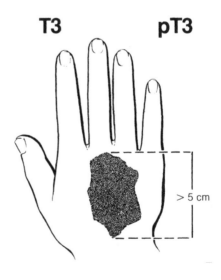

Fig. 252

T4   Tumour invades deep extradermal structures, i.e., cartilage, skeletal
            muscle, or bone (Fig. 253)

Note
In the case of multiple simultaneous tumours, the tumour with the highest T category is classified and the
number of separate tumours is indicated in parentheses, e.g., T2 (5) (Fig. 254)

T4   **pT4**   Fig. 253

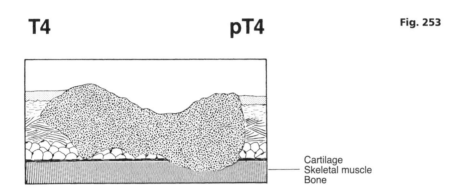

Cartilage
Skeletal muscle
Bone

T2(5)   **pT2**(5)   Fig. 254

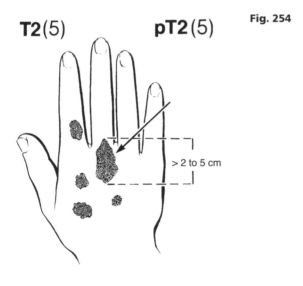

> 2 to 5 cm

N—Regional Lymph Nodes

NX   Regional lymph nodes cannot be assessed
N0   No regional lymph node metastasis
N1   Regional lymph node metastasis (Figs. 244–248, pp. 206–210)

M—Distant Metastasis

MX   Distant metastasis cannot be assessed
M0   No distant metastasis
M1   Distant metastasis (Figs. 244–248, pp. 206–210)

pTNM Pathological Classification

The pT, pN, and pM categories correspond to the T, N, and M categories.

pN0 Histological examination of a regional lymphadenectomy specimen will ordinarily include 6 or more lymph nodes. If the examined lymph nodes are negative, but the number ordinarily resected is not met, classify as pN0.

Summary

Skin Carcinoma	
T1	≤2 cm
T2	>2 to 5 cm
T3	>5 cm
T4	Deep extradermal structures (cartilage, skeletal muscle, bone)
N1	Regional

Malignant Melanoma of Skin

(ICD-O C44, C51.0, C60.9, C63.2)

Rules for Classification

There should be histological confirmation of the disease.

Regional Lymph Nodes

The regional lymph nodes are those appropriate to the site of the primary tumour. (See p. 204)

TNM Clinical Classification

T—Primary Tumour

The extent of the tumour is classified after excision, see pT, pp. 225–227.

N—Regional Lymph Nodes

NX   Regional lymph nodes cannot be assessed
N0   No regional lymph node metastasis

N1   Metastasis in one regional lymph node
    N1a   Only microscopic metastasis (clinically occult) (Fig. 255)
    N1b   Macroscopic metastasis (clinically apparent) (Fig. 256)
N2   Metastasis in two or three regional lymph nodes or satellites or in-transit metastasis
    N2a   Only microscopic metastasis (Fig. 257)
    N2b   Macroscopic metastasis (Fig. 258)
    N2c   Satellite or in-transit metastasis *without* regional lymph node metastasis (Figs. 259, 260)
N3   Metastasis in four or more regional lymph nodes (Fig. 261), or matted metastatic regional lymph nodes (Fig. 262), or satellite(s) or in-transit metastasis *with* metastasis in regional lymph node(s) (Figs. 263, 264)

Note

Satellites are tumour nests or nodules (macroscopic or microscopic) within 2 cm of the primary tumour. In-transit metastasis involves skin or subcutaneous tissue more than 2 cm from the primary tumour but not beyond the regional lymph nodes.

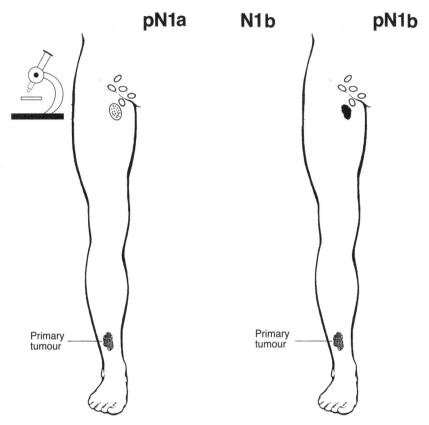

pN1a   **N1b**   **pN1b**

Primary tumour

Primary tumour

Fig. 255   **Fig. 256**

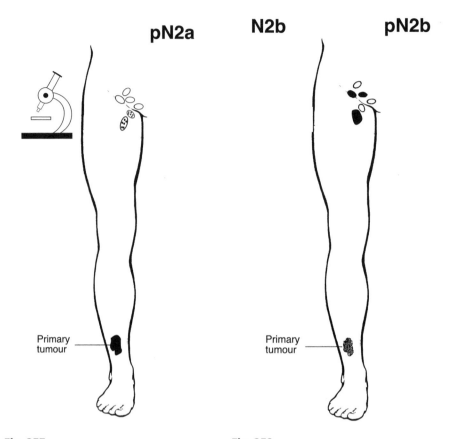

pN2a

N2b

pN2b

Primary
tumour

Primary
tumour

Fig. 257   **Fig. 258**

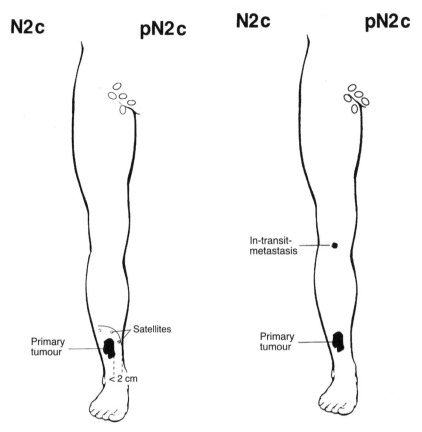

N2c   **pN2c**   **N2c**   **pN2c**

Satellites

Primary tumour

< 2 cm

In-transit-metastasis

Primary tumour

Fig. 259   **Fig. 260**

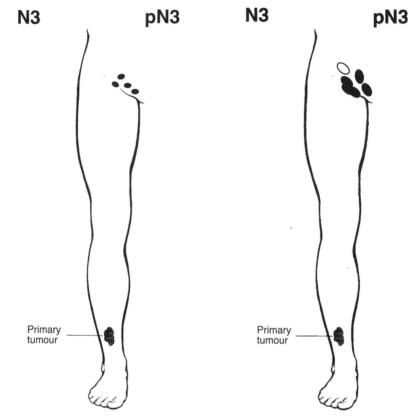

Fig. 261   Fig. 262

N3   **pN3**   Fig. 263

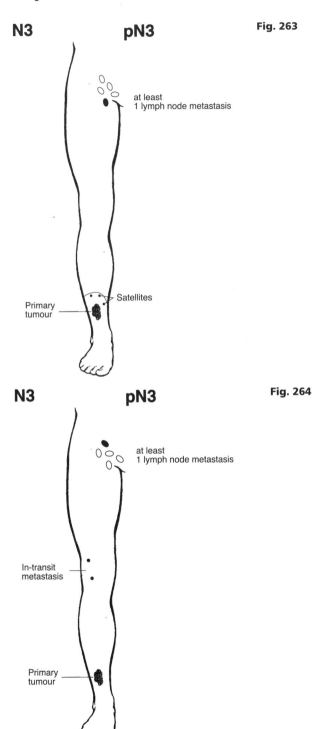

at least
1 lymph node metastasis

Satellites

Primary
tumour

N3   **pN3**   Fig. 264

at least
1 lymph node metastasis

In-transit
metastasis

Primary
tumour

M—Distant Metastasis

MX   Distant metastasis cannot be assessed
M0   No distant metastasis
M1   Distant metastasis
    M1a   Metastasis in skin or subcutaneous tissue or lymph node(s) beyond the
         regional lymph nodes (Fig. 244–247, pp. 206–209)
    M1b   Lung metastasis
    M1c   Metastasis in other sites, or any site and an elevated serum lactate
         dehydrogenase (LDH)

pTNM Pathological Classification

pT—Primary Tumour

Introductory Note

The pT classification of malignant melanoma considers three histological criteria:

1. Tumour thickness (Breslow) according to the largest vertical diameter of the
   tumour in millimeters (Fig. 265a, b)
2. Clark "levels" (Fig. 266)
3. Absence or presence of ulceration of the primary tumour (Fig. 265a, b)

The definitive pT category is based on these three criteria.

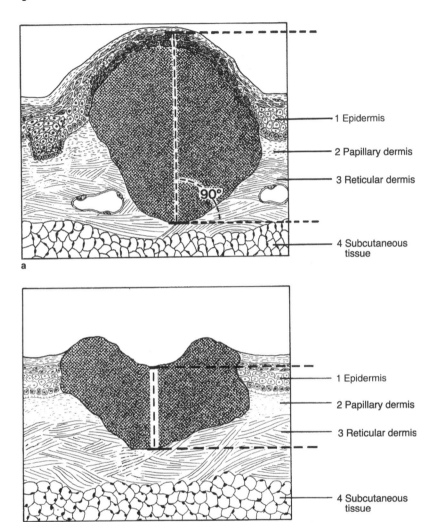

1 Epidermis

2 Papillary dermis

3 Reticular dermis

4 Subcutaneous tissue

1 Epidermis

2 Papillary dermis

3 Reticular dermis

4 Subcutaneous tissue

Fig. 265a, b

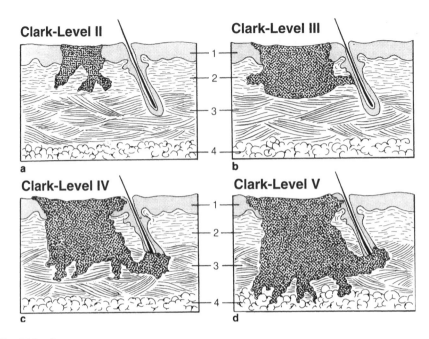

Fig. 266a-d

pT—Primary Tumour

pTX   Primary tumour cannot be assessed*
pT0   No evidence of primary tumour
pTis   Melanoma in situ (Clark level I) (atypical melanocytic hyperplasia, severe melanocytic
           dysplasia, not an invasive malignant lesion)

Note
pTX includes shave biopsies and regressed melanomas.

pT1   Tumour 1 mm or less in thickness (Fig. 267)
       pT1a   Clark level II or III, without ulceration
       pT1b   Clark level IV or V, or with ulceration
pT2   Tumour more than 1 mm but not more than 2 mm in thickness (Fig. 268)
       pT2a   Without ulceration
       pT2b   With ulceration
pT3   Tumour more than 2 mm but not more than 4 mm in thickness (Fig. 269)
       pT3a   Without ulceration
       pT3b   With ulceration

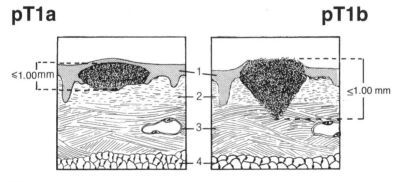

pT1a

pT1b

Fig. 267

pT2a   pT2b

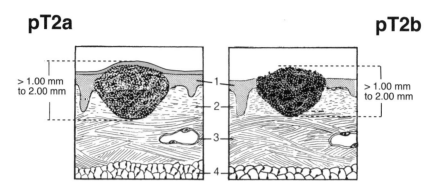

> 1.00 mm to 2.00 mm

> 1.00 mm to 2.00 mm

Fig. 268

pT3a   pT3b

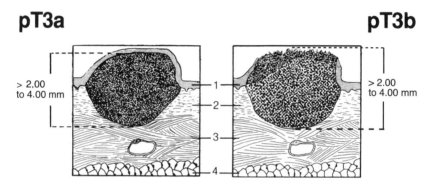

> 2.00 to 4.00 mm

> 2.00 to 4.00 mm

Fig. 269

pT4   Tumour more than 4 mm in thickness (Fig. 270)
        pT4a   Without ulceration
        pT4b   With ulceration

pT4a   pT4b

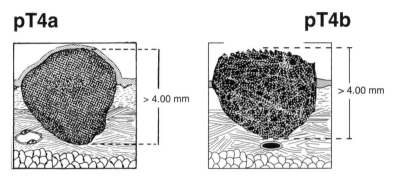

Fig. 270

pN—Regional Lymph Nodes

The pN categories correspond to the N categories (see Figs. 255–264, pp. 217–221).

pN0 Histological examination of a regional lymphadenectomy specimen will ordinarily include 6 or more lymph nodes. If the examined lymph nodes are negative, but the number ordinarily resected is not met, classify as pN0. Classification based solely on sentinel lymph node biopsy without subsequent axillary lymph node dissection is designated (sn) for sentinel lymph node, e.g., pN1(sn).

pM—Distant Metastasis

The pM categories correspond to the M categories.

Summary

Skin Malignant Melanoma	
pT1a	≤1 mm, Level II or III, no ulceration
pT1b	≤1 mm, Level IV or V, or ulceration
pT2a	>1–2 mm, no ulceration
pT2b	>1–2 mm, ulceration
pT3a	>2–4 mm, no ulceration
pT3b	>2–4 mm, ulceration
pT4a	>4 mm, no ulceration
pT4b	>4 mm, ulceration
N1	1 node
N1a	microscopic
N1b	macroscopic
N2	2–3 nodes or satellites/in-transit without nodes
N2a	2–3 nodes microscopic
N2b	2–3 nodes macroscopic
N2c	satellites or in-transit without nodes
N3	≥4 nodes; matted; satellites/in-transit with nodes

Breast Tumours (ICD-O C50)

Rules for Classification

The classification applies to carcinomas of the male as well as of the female breast. There should be histological confirmation of the disease. The anatomical subsite of origin should be recorded but is not considered in classification.

In the case of multiple simultaneous primary tumours in one breast, the tumour with the highest T category should be used for classification. Simultaneous *bilateral* breast cancers should be classified independently to permit division of cases by histological type.

TNM Atlas: Illustrated Guide to the TNM Classification of Malignant Tumours, Fifth Edition,
edited by Christian Wittekind, Frederick L. Greene, Robert Hutter, Martin Klimpfinger, and Leslie H. Sobin
Copyright © 2005 UICC

Anatomical Subsites (Fig. 271)

1. Nipple (C50.0)
2. Central portion (C50.1)
3. Upper-inner quadrant (C50.2)
4. Lower-inner quadrant (C50.3)
5. Upper-outer quadrant (C50.4)
6. Lower-outer quadrant (C50.5)
7. Axillary tail (C50.6)
8. Overlapping lesions (C50.8)

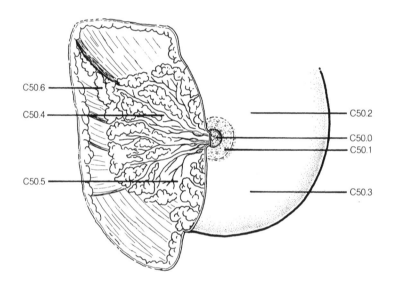

Fig. 271

Regional Lymph Nodes (Fig. 272)

The regional lymph nodes are:

1. *Axillary* (ipsilateral): interpectoral (Rotter) nodes and lymph nodes along the axillary vein and its tributaries, which may be divided into the following levels:
   (i) *Level I* (low-axilla): lymph nodes lateral to the lateral border of pectoralis minor muscle.
   (ii) *Level II* (mid-axilla): lymph nodes between the medial and lateral borders of the pectoralis minor muscle and the interpectoral (Rotter) lymph nodes.
   (iii) *Level III* (apical axilla): lymph nodes medial to the medial margin of the pectoralis minor muscle, excluding those designated as subclavicular or infraclavicular.

Note
Intramammary lymph nodes are coded as axillary lymph nodes.

2. *Infraclavicular* (subclavicular) (ipsilateral).
3. *Internal mammary* (ipsilateral): lymph nodes in the intercostal spaces along the edge of the sternum in the endothoracic fascia.
4. *Supraclavicular* (ipsilateral).

Any other lymph node metastasis is coded as a distant metastasis (M1), including, cervical, or contralateral internal mammary lymph nodes.

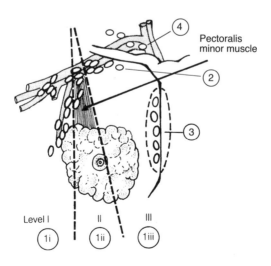

Fig. 272

TN Clinical Classification

T—Primary Tumour

TX   Primary tumour cannot be assessed
T0   No evidence of primary tumour
Tis   Carcinoma in situ

Tis (DCIS)   Ductal carcinoma in situ
Tis (LCIS)   Lobular carcinoma in situ
Tis (Paget)   Paget disease of the nipple with no tumour (Fig. 273)

Note
Paget disease associated with a tumour is classified according to the size of the tumour.

T1   Tumour 2.0 cm or less in greatest dimension
          T1mic   Microinvasion 0.1 cm or less in greatest dimension[1] (Fig. 274)
          T1a   More than 0.1 cm but not more than 0.5 cm in greatest dimension
                  (Fig. 275)
          T1b   More than 0.5 cm but not more than 1.0 cm in greatest dimension
                  (Fig. 275)
          T1c   More than 1.0 cm but not more than 2.0 cm in greatest dimension
                  (Fig. 275)
T2   Tumour more than 2.0 cm but not more than 5.0 cm in greatest
          dimension (Fig. 276)

Note
[1] Microinvasion is the extension of cancer cells beyond the basement membrane into the adjacent tissue with no focus more than 0.1 cm in greatest dimension. When there are multiple foci of microinvasion, the size of only the largest focus is used to classify the microinvasion. (Do not use the sum of all individual foci.) The presence of multiple foci of microinvasion should be noted, as it is with multiple larger invasive carcinomas (Fig. 274).

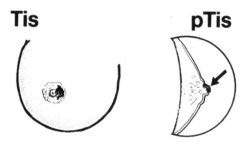

Fig. 273

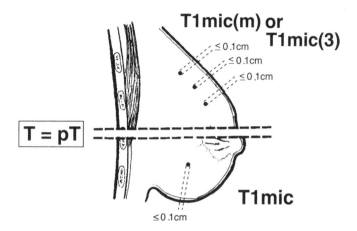

Fig. 274

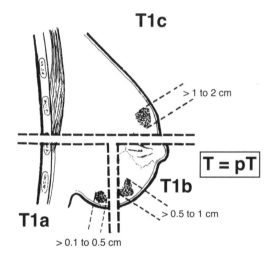

Fig. 275

T3   Tumour more than 5 cm in greatest dimension (Fig. 276)

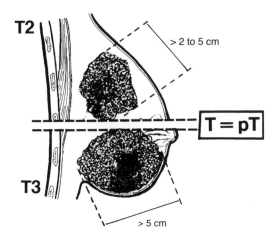

Fig. 276

T4 Tumour of any size with direct extension to chest wall or skin only as described in T4a to T4d

T4a Extension to chest wall[2] (Fig. 277)

T4b Oedema (including peau d'orange), or ulceration of the skin of the breast, or satellite skin nodules confined to the same breast (Figs. 278, 279)

T4c Both 4a and 4b, above (Fig. 280)

T4d Inflammatory carcinoma[3] (Fig. 281)

Notes

[2] Chest wall includes ribs, intercostal muscles, and serratus anterior muscle but not pectoral muscle

[3] Inflammatory carcinoma of the breast is characterized by diffuse, brawny induration of the skin with an erysipeloid edge, usually with no underlying mass. If the skin biopsy is negative and there is no localized measurable primary cancer, the T category is pTX when pathologically staging a clinical inflammatory carcinoma (T4d). Dimpling of the skin, nipple retraction, or other skin changes, except those in T4b and T4d, may occur in T1, T2, or T3 without affecting the classification.

T4a   pT4a

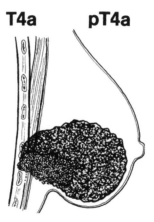

Fig. 277

T4b   pT4b

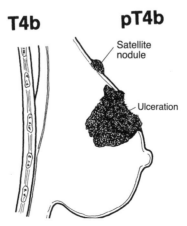

Satellite nodule

Ulceration

Fig. 278

T4b   **pT4b**   Fig. 279

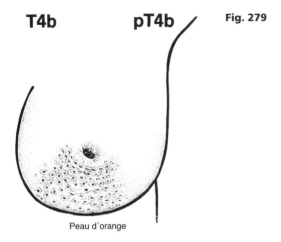

Peau d´orange

T4c   **pT4c**   Fig. 280

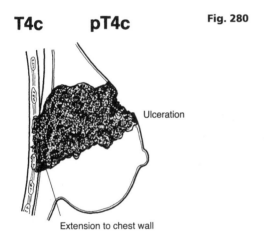

Ulceration

Extension to chest wall

T4d   **pT4d**   Fig. 281

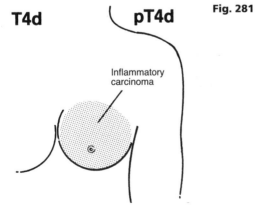

Inflammatory
carcinoma

N—Regional Lymph Nodes

NX   Regional lymph nodes cannot be assessed (e.g., previously removed)

N0   No regional lymph node metastasis

N1   Metastasis into movable ipsilateral axillary node(s) (Fig. 282)

N2   Metastasis in fixed ipsilateral axillary lymph node(s) or in clinically apparent* ipsilateral internal mammary lymph node(s) in the absence of clinically evident axillary lymph node metastasis

    N2a   Metastasis in ipsilateral axillary lymph node(s) fixed to one another or to other structures (Fig. 283)

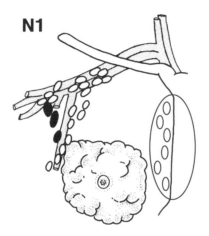

Fig. 282

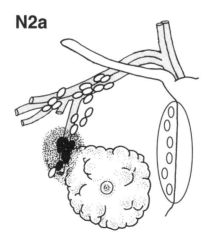

Fig. 283

N2b   Metastasis only in clinically apparent* ipsilateral internal mammary
       lymph node(s) and in the absence of clinically evident ipsilateral
       axillary lymph node metastasis (Fig. 284)
N3   Metastasis in ipsilateral infraclavicular lymph node(s) with or without
      axillary lymph node(s); or in clinically apparent* ipsilateral internal
      mammary lymph node(s) and when occurring in the presence of clinically
      evident axillary lymph node metastasis; or metastasis in ipsilateral
      supraclavicular lymph node(s) with or without axillary or internal
      mammary lymph node involvement

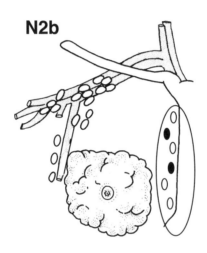

N2b

Fig. 284

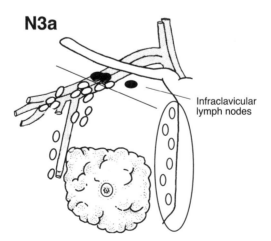

N3a

Infraclavicular
lymph nodes

Fig. 285

Breast Tumours

N3a   Metastasis in ipsilateral infraclavicular lymph node(s) (Fig. 285)

N3b   Metastasis in ipsilateral internal mammary and axillary lymph nodes (Fig. 286)

N3c   Metastasis in ipsilateral supraclavicular lymph node(s) (Fig. 287)

Note

* Clinically apparent = detected by imaging studies (excluding lymphoscintigraphy) or by clinical examination

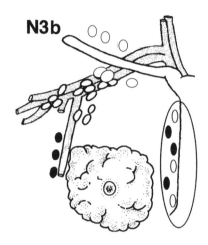

Fig. 286

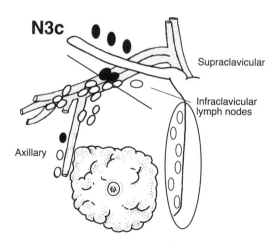

Fig. 287

pTNM Pathological Classification

pT—Primary Tumour

The pathological classification requires the examination of the primary carcinoma with no gross tumour at the margins of resection. A case can be classified pT if there is only microscopic tumour in a margin.

The pT category corresponds to the T category.

Note

When classifying pT the tumour size is a measurement of the invasive component. If there is a large in situ component (e.g., 4.0 cm) and a small invasive component (e.g., 0.5 cm), the tumour is coded pT1a.

pN—Regional Lymph Nodes

The pathological classification requires the resection and examination of at least the low axillary lymph nodes (level I) (see page 231). Such a resection will ordinarily include 6 or more lymph nodes. If the examined lymph nodes are negative, but the number ordinarily resected is not met, classify as pN0.

Examination of one or more sentinel lymph nodes may be used for pathological classification. If classification is based solely on sentinel lymph node biopsy without subsequent axillary lymph node dissection it should be designated (sn) for sentinel lymph node, e.g., pN1(sn).

pNX   Regional lymph nodes cannot be assessed (not removed for study or
        previously removed)

pN0   No regional lymph node metastasis

Note

Cases with only isolated tumour cells (ITC) in regional lymph nodes are classified as pN0. ITC are single tumour cells or small clusters of cells, not more than 0.2 mm in greatest dimension, that are usually detected by immunohistochemistry or molecular methods but which may be verified on H&E stains. ITC do not typically show evidence of metastatic activity, e.g., proliferation or stromal reaction.

pN1(mi) Micrometastasis (greater than 0.2 mm but not more than 2.0 mm in greatest dimension) (Fig. 288)

pN1 Metastasis in 1 to 3 ipsilateral axillary lymph node(s), and/or ipsilateral internal mammary lymph nodes with microscopic metastasis detected by sentinel lymph node dissection but not clinically apparent**

   pN1a Metastasis in 1 to 3 axillary lymph node(s), including at least one larger than 2 mm in greatest dimension (Fig. 289)

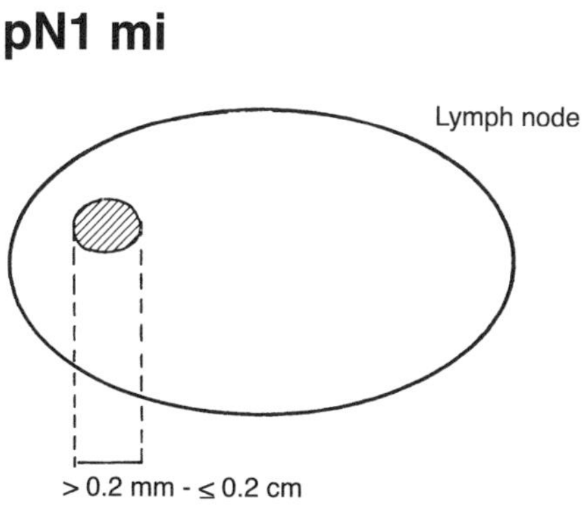

pN1 mi

Fig. 288

Lymph node

> 0.2 mm - ≤ 0.2 cm

pN1a

Fig. 289

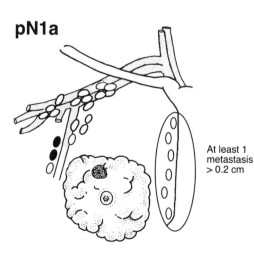

At least 1
metastasis
> 0.2 cm

pN1b Internal mammary lymph nodes with microscopic metastasis
       detected by sentinel lymph node dissection but not clinically
       apparent** (Fig. 290)
pN1c Metastasis in 1 to 3 axillary lymph nodes and in internal mammary
       lymph nodes with microscopic metastasis detected by sentinel
       lymph node dissection but not clinically apparent** (Fig. 291)

pN1b

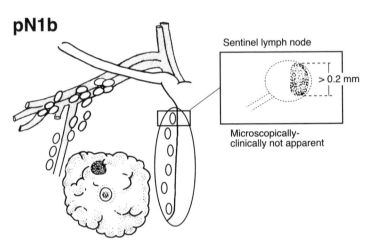

Fig. 290

pN1c

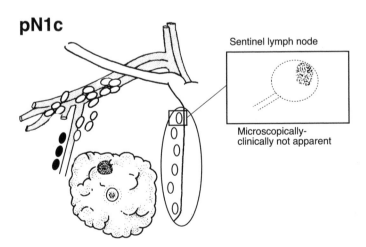

Fig. 291

pN2   Metastasis into 4 to 9 ipsilateral axillary lymph nodes, or in clinically apparent** internal mammary lymph node(s) in the absence of axillary lymph node metastasis

pN2a Metastasis into 4 to 9 axillary lymph nodes, including at least one that is larger than 2 mm in greatest dimension (Fig. 292)

pN2b Metastasis in clinically apparent** internal mammary lymph node(s), in the *absence* of axillary lymph node metastasis (Fig. 293)

pN2a

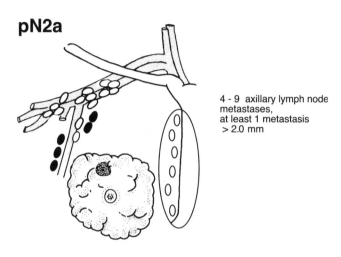

4 - 9 axillary lymph node metastases,
at least 1 metastasis
> 2.0 mm

Fig. 292

pN2b

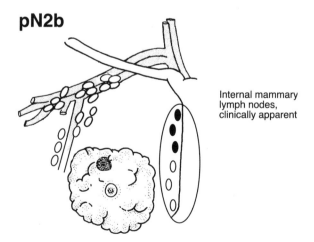

Internal mammary lymph nodes,
clinically apparent

Fig. 293

pN3   Metastasis in 10 or more ipsilateral axillary lymph nodes; or in
       ipsilateral infraclavicular lymph nodes; or in clinically apparent**
       ipsilateral internal mammary lymph nodes in the *presence* of one or
       more positive axillary lymph nodes; or in more than 3 axillary lymph
       nodes with clinically negative, microscopic metastasis in internal
       mammary lymph nodes; or in ipsilateral supraclavicular lymph nodes
       pN3a Metastasis in 10 or more axillary lymph nodes (at least one larger
            than 2 mm in greatest dimension) or metastasis in infraclavicular
            lymph nodes (Figs. 294, 295)

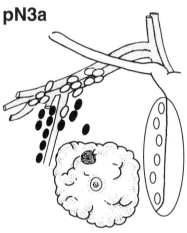

pN3a

Fig. 294

≥ 10 axillary lymph node metastasis,
at least one metastasis > 2.0 cm

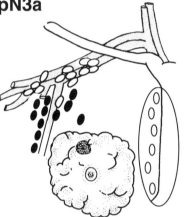

pN3a

Fig. 295

pN3b Metastasis in clinically apparent* internal mammary lymph
node(s) in the *presence* of one or more positive axillary lymph
node(s) (Fig. 296); or metastasis in more than 3 axillary lymph
nodes *and* in internal mammary lymph nodes with microscopic
metastasis detected by sentinel lymph node dissection but not
clinically apparent**

pN3c Metastasis in supraclavicular lymph nodes (Fig. 297)

Note

* not clinically apparent = not detected by clinical examination or by imaging studies (excluding lymphoscintigraphy)

** clinically apparent: detected by clinical examination or by imaging studies (excluding lymphoscintigraphy) or grossly visible pathologically.

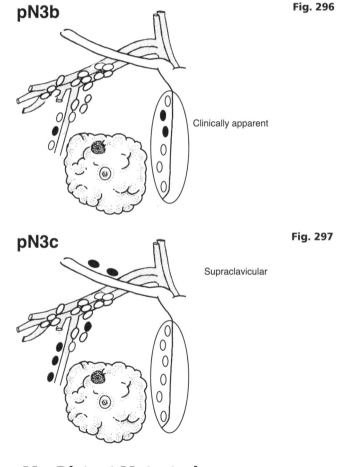

pN3b

Fig. 296

Clinically apparent

pN3c

Fig. 297

Supraclavicular

pM—Distant Metastasis

The pM categories correspond to the M categories.

Summary

Breast			
Tis	In situ		
T1	≤2 cm		
T1mic	≤0.1 cm		
T1a	>0.1 to 0.5 cm		
T1b	>0.5 to 1 cm		
T1c	>1 to 2 cm		
T2	>2 to 5 cm		
T3	>5 cm		
T4	Chest wall/skin		
T4a	Chest wall		
T4b	Skin oedema/ulceration, satellite skin nodules		
T4c	Both 4a and 4b		
T4d	Inflammatory carcinoma		
N1	Movable axillary	pN1mi	Micrometastasis, >0.2 mm ≤2 mm
		pN1a	1–3 axillary nodes
		pN1b	Internal mammary nodes with microscopic metastasis by sentinal node biopsy but not clinically apparent
		pN1c	1–3 axillary nodes and internal mammary nodes with microscopic metastasis by sentinal node biopsy but not clinically apparent
N2a	Fixed axillary	pN2a	4–9 axillary nodes
N2b	Internal mammary clinically apparent	pN2b	Internal mammary nodes, clinically apparent, without axillary nodes
N3a	Infraclavicular	pN3a	≥10 axillary nodes or infraclavicular node(s)
N3b	Internal mammary and axillary	pN3b	Internal mammary nodes, clinically apparent, with axillary node(s) or >3 axillary nodes and internal mammary nodes with microscopic metastasis by sentinal node biopsy but not clinically apparent
N3c	Supraclavicular	pN3c	Supraclavicular

Gynaecological Tumours

Introductory Notes

The following sites are included:

- Vulva
- Vagina
- Cervix uteri
- Corpus uteri
- Ovary
- Fallopian tube
- Gestational trophoblastic tumours

Cervix uteri and corpus uteri were amongst the first sites to be classified by the TNM system. The "League of Nations" stages for carcinoma of the cervix have been used with minor modifications for over 50 years, and, because these are accepted by the Fédération Internationale de Gynécologie et d'Obstétrique (FIGO), the TNM categories have been defined to correspond to the FIGO stages. Some amendments have been made in collaboration with FIGO, and the classifications now published have the approval of the FIGO, UICC, and the national TNM committees including the AJCC.

TNM Atlas: Illustrated Guide to the TNM Classification of Malignant Tumours, Fifth Edition,
edited by Christian Wittekind, Frederick L. Greene, Robert Hutter, Martin Klimpfinger, and Leslie H. Sobin
Copyright © 2005 UICC

Vulva (ICD-O C51)

The definitions of the T, N, and M categories correspond to FIGO stages. Both systems are included for comparison.

Rules for Classification

The classification applies only to primary carcinomas of the vulva. There should be histological confirmation of the disease.

A carcinoma of the vulva that has extended to the vagina is classified as carcinoma of the vulva.

The FIGO stages are based on surgical staging. TNM stages are based on clinical and/or pathological classification.

Anatomical Subsites (Fig. 298)

1. Labia majora (C51.0)
2. Labia minora (C51.1)
3. Clitoris (C51.2)

Regional Lymph Nodes

The regional lymph nodes are the femoral and inguinal nodes.

Fig. 298

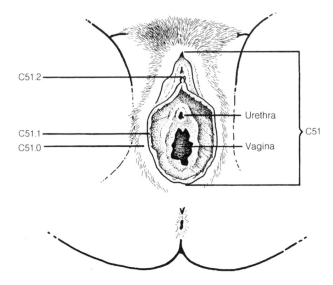

C51.2

C51.1

C51.0

Urethra

Vagina

C51

TNM Clinical Classification

T—Primary Tumour

TX   Primary tumour cannot be assessed
T0   No evidence of primary tumour
Tis   Carcinoma in situ (preinvasive carcinoma)

T1   Tumour confined to vulva or vulva and perineum, 2.0 cm or less in greatest dimension (Fig. 299)

        T1a   Tumour confined to vulva or vulva and perineum, 2.0 cm or less in greatest dimension and with stromal invasion no greater than 1.0 mm* (Fig. 300a)

        T1b   Tumour confined to vulva or vulva and perineum, 2.0 cm or less in greatest dimension and with stromal invasion greater than 1.0 mm* (Fig. 300b)

Note

* The depth of invasion is defined as the measurement of the tumour from the epithelial-stromal junction of the adjacent most superficial dermal papilla to the deepest point of invasion.

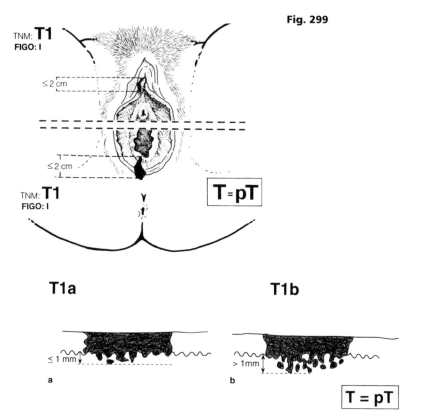

Fig. 299

TNM: **T1**
FIGO: I

≤ 2 cm

≤ 2 cm

TNM: **T1**
FIGO: I

$T = pT$

T1a

T1b

≤ 1 mm

\> 1 mm

a

b

$T = pT$

Fig. 300a, b

T2   Tumour confined to vulva or vulva and perineum, more than 2.0 cm in
      greatest dimension (Fig. 301)
T3   Tumour invades any of the following: lower urethra, vagina, anus
      (Figs. 302, 303)

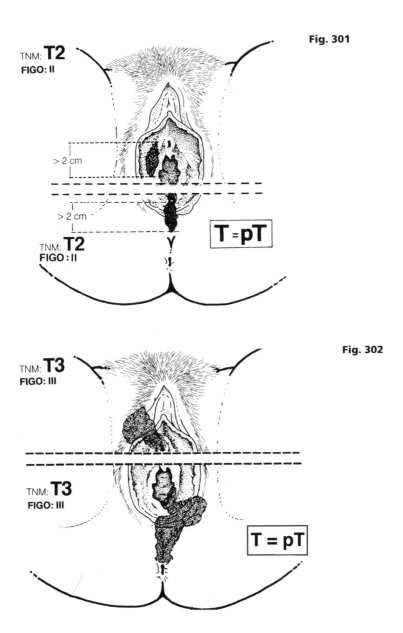

Fig. 301

TNM: **T2**
FIGO: II

> 2 cm

> 2 cm

T = pT

TNM: **T2**
FIGO : II

Fig. 302

TNM: **T3**
FIGO: III

TNM: **T3**
FIGO: III

T = pT

T4   Tumour invades any of the following: bladder mucosa, rectal mucosa, upper urethral mucosa; or is fixed to pubic bone (Fig. 304)

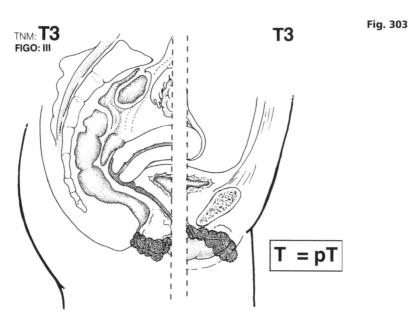

Fig. 303

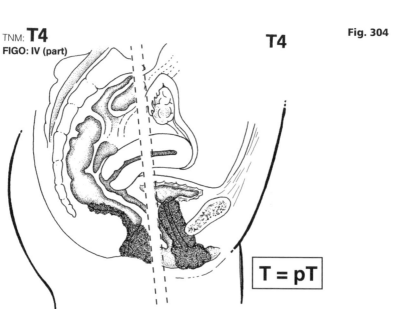

Fig. 304

N—Regional Lymph Nodes

NX   Regional lymph nodes cannot be assessed
N0   No regional lymph node metastasis
N1   Unilateral regional lymph node metastasis (Fig. 305)
N2   Bilateral regional lymph node metastasis (Fig. 306)

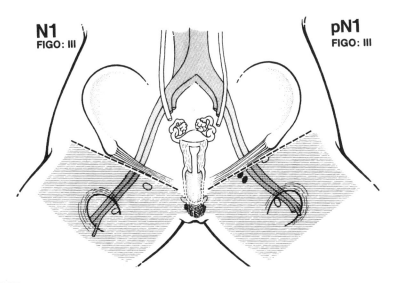

Fig. 305

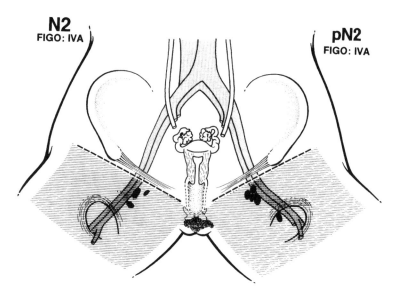

Fig. 306

pTN Pathological Classification

The pT and pN categories correspond to the T and N categories.

pN0 Histological examination of an inguinal lymphadenectomy specimen will ordinarily include 6 or more lymph nodes.

If the examined lymph nodes are negative, but the number ordinarily resected is not met, classify as pN0.

Summary

TNM	Vulva	FIGO
T1	Confined to vulva/perineum ≤2 cm	I
T1a	Stromal invasion ≤1.0 mm	IA
T1b	Stromal invasion >1.0 mm	IB
T2	Confined to vulva/perineum >2 cm	II
T3	Lower urethra/vagina/anus	III
T4	Bladder mucosa/rectal mucosa/upper urethra/bone	IVA
N1	Unilateral	III
N2	Bilateral	IVA
M1	Distant metastasis	IVB

Vagina (ICD-O C52) (Fig. 307)

The definitions of the T and M categories correspond to the FIGO stages. Both systems are included for comparison.

The FIGO stages are based on surgical staging. (TNM stages are based on clinical and/or pathological classification).

Rules for Classification

The classification applies to primary carcinomas only.

Tumours present in the vagina as secondary growths from either genital or extragenital sites are excluded.

A tumour that has extended to the portio and reached the external os (orifice of uterus) is classified as carcinoma of the cervix.

A tumour involving the vulva is classified as carcinoma of the vulva.

Fig. 307

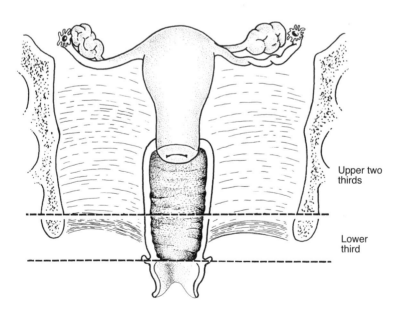

Upper two thirds

Lower third

Regional Lymph Nodes

Upper two-thirds of vagina:

The pelvic nodes including obturator, internal iliac (hypogastric), external iliac, and pelvic nodes, NOS (Fig. 308).

Lower third of vagina:

The inguinal nodes and femoral nodes (Fig. 309).

Fig. 308

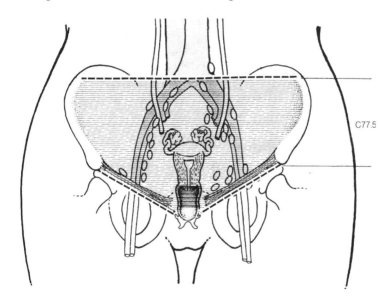

C77.5

Fig. 309

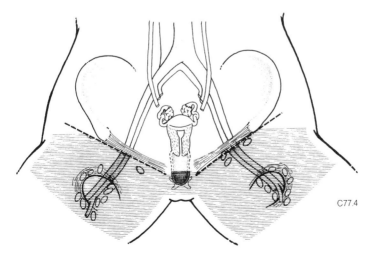

C77.4

Vagina

TNM Clinical Classification

T—Primary Tumour

TNM Categories	FIGO stages	
TX		Primary tumour cannot be assessed
T0		No evidence of primary tumour
Tis		Carcinoma in situ (preinvasive carcinoma)
T1	I	Tumour confined to vagina (Fig. 310)
T2	II	Tumour invades paravaginal tissues but does not extend to pelvic wall (Fig. 311)
T3	III	Tumour extends to pelvic wall (Fig. 312)
T4	IVA	Tumour invades mucosa of the bladder or rectum and/or extends beyond the true pelvis (Fig. 313)
M1	IVB	Distant metastasis

Note

The presence of bullous oedema is not sufficient evidence to classify a tumour as T4.

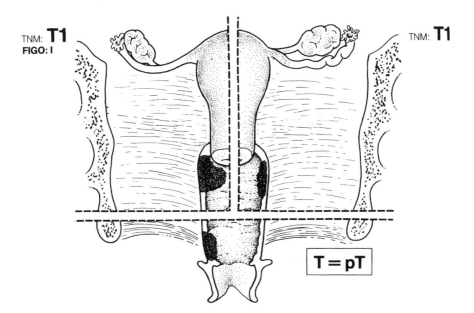

TNM: **T1**
FIGO: I

TNM: **T1**

T = pT

Fig. 310

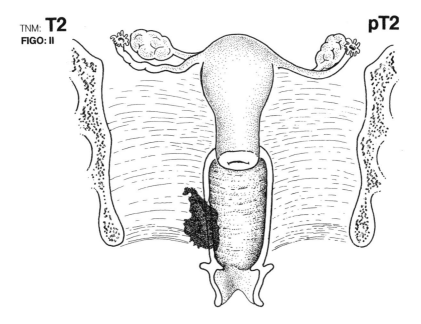

TNM: **T2**
FIGO: II

pT2

Fig. 311

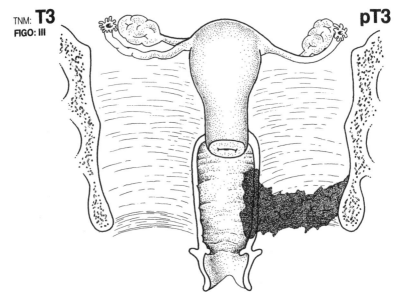

TNM: **T3**
FIGO: III

pT3

Fig. 312

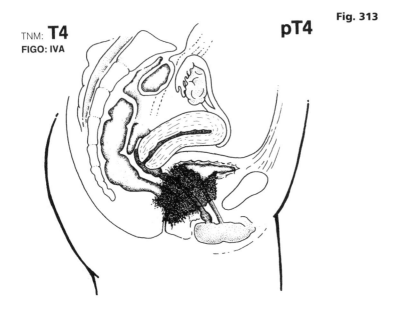

Fig. 313

TNM: **T4**
FIGO: IVA

pT4

N—Regional Lymph Nodes

NX   Regional lymph nodes cannot be assessed
N0   No regional lymph node metastasis
N1   Regional lymph node metastasis (Figs. 314–316)

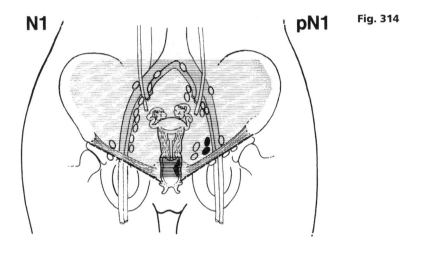

Fig. 314

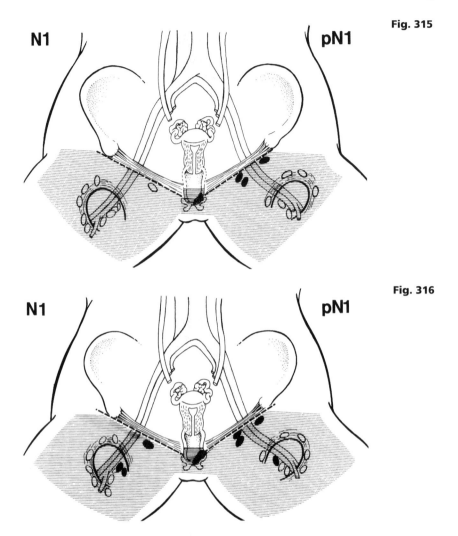

Fig. 315

Fig. 316

pTN Pathological Classification

The pT and pN categories correspond to the T and N categories.

pN0 Histological examination of an inguinal lymphadenectomy specimen will ordinarily include 6 or more lymph nodes; a pelvic lymphadenectomy specimen will ordinarily include 10 or more lymph nodes.

If the examined lymph nodes are negative, but the number ordinarily resected is not met, classify as pN0.

Summary

TNM	Vagina	FIGO
T1	Vaginal wall	I
T2	Paravaginal tissue	II
T3	Extends to pelvic wall	III
T4	Mucosa of bladder/rectum, beyond pelvis	IVA
N1	Regional	—
M1	Distant metastasis	IVB

Cervix Uteri (ICD-O C53)

The definitions of the T and M categories correspond to the FIGO stages. Both systems are included for comparison.

The FIGO stages are based on surgical staging. This includes histological examination of a cone of amputation of the cervix. (TNM stages are based on clinical and/or pathological classification.)

Rules for Classification

The classification applies only to carcinomas. There should be histological confirmation of the disease.

Anatomical Subsites (Fig. 317)

1. Endocervix (C53.0)
2. Exocervix (C53.1)

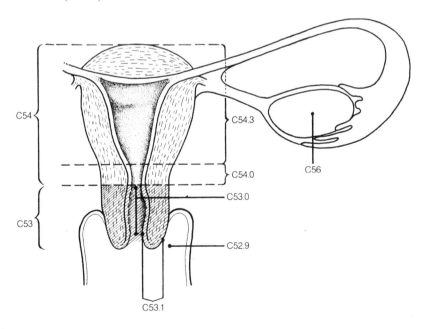

Fig. 317

Regional Lymph Nodes (Fig. 318)

The regional lymph nodes are:

(1) paracervical nodes
(2) parametrial nodes
(3) hypogastric (internal iliac) including obturator nodes
(4) external iliac nodes
(5) common iliac nodes
(6) presacral nodes
(7) lateral sacral nodes (not shown in Fig. 318)

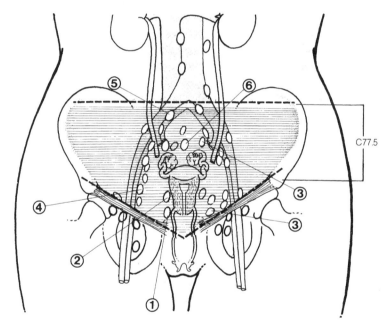

Fig. 318

TNM Clinical Classification

T—Primary Tumour

TNM Categories	FIGO stages	
TX		Primary tumour cannot be assessed
T0		No evidence of primary tumour
Tis		Carcinoma in situ (preinvasive carcinoma)
T1	I	Cervical carcinoma confined to uterus (extension to corpus should be disregarded)
T1a	IA	Invasive carcinoma diagnosed only by microscopy. All macroscopically visible lesions—even with superficial invasion—are T1b/Stage IB (Fig. 319)
T1a1	IA1	Stromal invasion no greater than 3.0 mm in depth and 7.0 mm or less in horizontal spread (Fig. 320)
T1a2	IA2	Stromal invasion more than 3.0 mm and not more than 5.0 mm with a horizontal spread 7.0 mm or less (Fig. 321)

Note

The depth of invasion should not be more than 5.0 mm taken from the base of the epithelium, either surface or glandular, from which it originates. The depth of invasion is defined as the measurement of the tumour from the epithelial-stromal junction of the adjacent most superficial epithelial papilla to the deepest point of invasion.

T1b	IB	Clinically visible lesion confined to the cervix (Figs. 322, 324) or microscopic lesion greater than T1a2/IA2 (Fig. 323)*
T1b1	IB1	Clinically visible lesion 4.0 cm or less in greatest dimension (Fig. 322)
T1b2	IB2	Clinically visible lesion more than 4.0 cm in greatest dimension (Fig. 324)
T2	II	Tumor invades beyond uterus but not to pelvic wall or to lower third of the vagina (Fig. 325)
T2a	IIA	Without parametrial invasion
T2b	IIB	With parametrial invasion

*Note

Lesions diagnosed only by microscopy greater than T1a2/IA2 should be classified as T1b1/IB1 (Fig. 323)

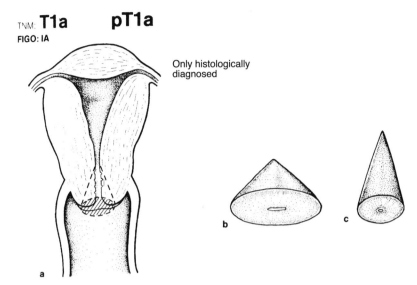

TNM: **T1a** **pT1a**
FIGO: IA

Only histologically
diagnosed

a

b

c

Fig. 319a-c

TNM: **T1a1**   **pT1a1**
FIGO: IA1

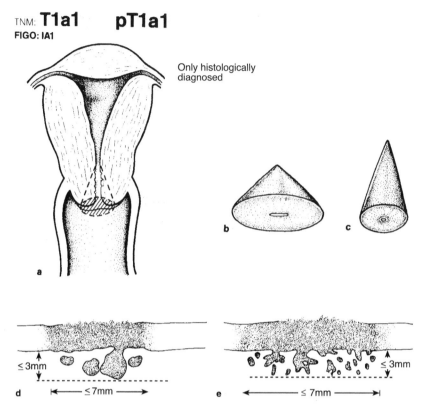

Only histologically
diagnosed

Fig. 320a-e

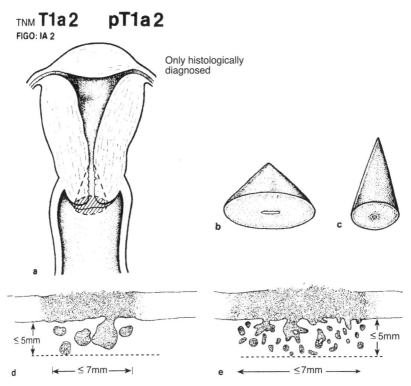

TNM **T1a2**   **pT1a2**

FIGO: IA 2

Only histologically diagnosed

Fig. 321a-c

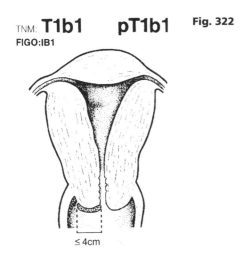

TNM: **T1b1**   **pT1b1**   Fig. 322

FIGO:IB1

≤4cm

TNM: **T1b1**
FIGO: IB1

pT1b1

Only histologically
diagnosed

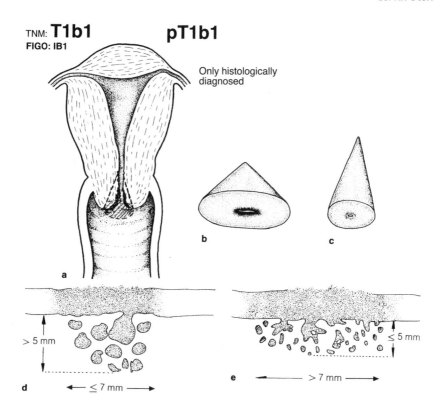

Fig. 323a-e

TNM: **T1b2**
FIGO: IB2

pT1b2

Fig. 324

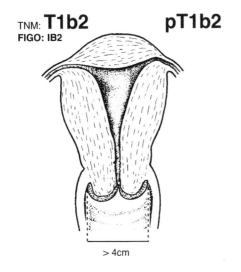

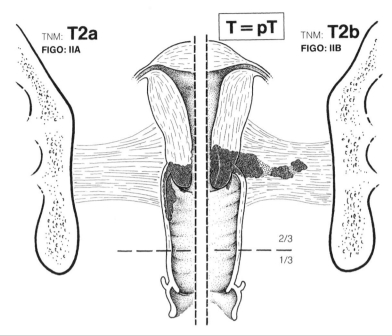

TNM: **T2a**
FIGO: IIA

T = pT

TNM: **T2b**
FIGO: IIB

2/3

1/3

Fig. 325

TNM Categories	FIGO stages	
T3	III	Tumor extends to pelvic wall and/or involves the lower third of vagina and/or causes hydronephrosis or non-functioning kidney (Fig. 326)
T3a	IIIA	Tumor involves lower third of vagina, no extension to pelvic wall
T3b	IIIB	Tumor extend to pelvic wall and/or causes hydronephrosis or non-functioning kidney
T4	IVA	Tumor invades mucosa of bladder or rectum and/or extend beyond true pelvis (Fig. 327)

Note
The presence of bullous oedema is not sufficient evidence to classify a tumour as T4. Invasion of bladder and rectum mucosa should by biopsy proven.

M1	IVB	Distant metastasis

Fig. 326

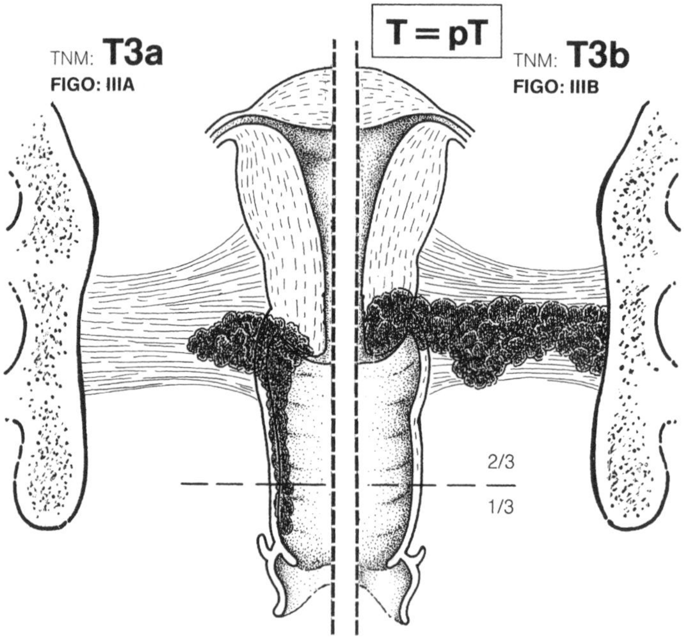

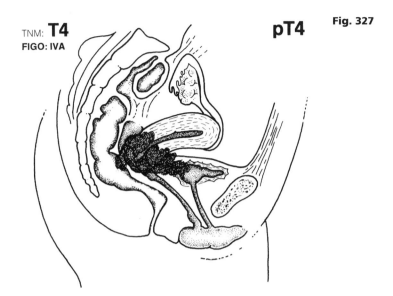

Fig. 327

TNM: **T4**
FIGO: **IVA**

pT4

N—Regional Lymph Nodes

NX   Regional lymph nodes cannot be assessed
N0   No regional lymph node metastasis
N1   Regional lymph node metastasis (Fig. 328)

pTNM Pathological Classification

The pT, pN, and pM categories correspond to the T, N, and M categories.

pN0 Histological examination of a pelvic lymphadenectomy specimen will ordinarily include 10 or more lymph nodes.

If the examined lymph nodes are negative, but the number ordinarily resected is not met, classify as pN0.

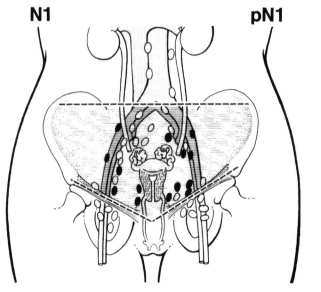

Fig. 328

N1   pN1

Summary

TNM	Cervix Uteri	FIGO
Tis	In situ	0
T1	Confined to uterus	I
T1a	Diagnosed only by microscopy	IA
T1a1	Depth ≤3 mm, horizontal spread ≤7 mm	IA1
T1a2	Depth >3–5 mm, horizontal spread ≤7 mm	IA2
T1b	Clinically visible or microscopic lesion, greater than T1a2	IB
T1b1	≤4 cm	IB1
T1b2	>4 cm	IB2
T2	Beyond uterus but not pelvic wall or lower third vagina	II
T2a	No parametrium	IIA
T2b	Parametrium	IIB
T3	Lower third vagina/pelvic wall/hydronephrosis	III
T3a	Lower third vagina	IIIA
T3b	Pelvic wall/hydronephrosis	IIIB
T4	Mucosa of bladder/rectum; beyond true pelvis	IVA
N1	Regional	—
M1	Distant metastasis	IVB

Corpus Uteri (ICD-O C54)

The definitions of the T, N, and M categories correspond to the FIGO stages. Both systems are included for comparison.

The FIGO stages are based on surgical staging. (TNM stages are based on clinical and/or pathological classification).

Rules for Classification

The classification applies only to carcinomas and malignant mixed mesodermal tumours. There should be histological verification with subdivision of histological type and grading of the carcinomas. The diagnosis should be based on examination of specimens taken by endometrial biopsy.

Editor's Note

FIGO does not recommend this classification for mixed mesodermal tumours.

The FIGO recommends that stage I patients given primary radiotherapy can be clinically classified as follows:

Stage I: Tumour limited to corpus uteri
Stage IA: Length of 8.0 cm or less
Stage IB: Length of more than 8.0 cm

Anatomical Subsites (Fig. 317, p. 264)

1. Isthmus uteri (C54.0)
2. Fundus uteri (C54.3)

Regional Lymph Nodes (Fig. 334, p. 283)

The regional lymph nodes are:

(1) the pelvic lymph nodes
   – hypogastric [obturator, internal iliac (1)]
   – common iliac (2)
   – external iliac (3)
   – parametrial (not shown in figures)
   – sacral (presacral, lateral sacral) (4)
   and
(2) the para-aortic lymph nodes including paracaval and interaortocaval lymph nodes (5).

TNM Clinical Classification

T—Primary Tumour

TNM Categories	FIGO Stages		
TX			Primary tumour cannot be assessed
T0			No evidence of primary tumour
Tis	0		Carcinoma in situ(preinvasive carcinoma)
T1	I		Tumour confined to corpus uteri (Fig. 329)
T1a		IA	Tumour limited to endometrium
T1b		IB	Tumour invades less than one half of myometrium
T1c		IC	Tumour invades one half or more of myometrium
T2	II		Tumour invades cervix but does not extend beyond uterus (Fig. 330)
T2a		IIA	Endocervical glandular involvement only
T2b		IIB	Cervical stromal invasion
T3 and/or N1	III		Local and/or regional spread as specified in T3a, b, N1, and FIGO IIIA, B, C below
T3a		IIIA	Tumour involves serosa and/or adnexa (direct extension or metastasis) and/or cancer cells in ascites or peritoneal washings (Fig. 331)
T3b		IIIB	Vaginal involvement (direct extension or metastasis) (Fig. 331)
N1		IIIC	Metastasis to pelvic and/or para-aortic lymph nodes (Fig. 333)
T4		IVA	Tumour invades bladder *mucosa* and/or bowel *mucosa* (Fig. 332)
			Note The presence of bullous edema is not sufficient evidence to classify a tumour as T4. The lesion should be confirmed by biopsy.
M1		IVB	Distant metastasis (*excluding* metastasis to vagina, pelvic serosa, or adnexa, *including* metastasis to intra-abdominal lymph nodes other than para-aortic, and/or pelvic nodes)

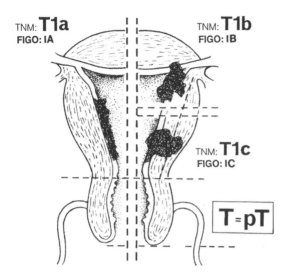

Fig. 329

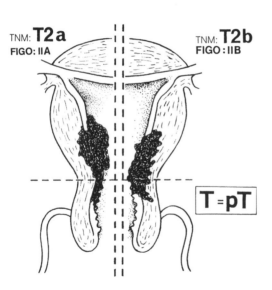

Fig. 330

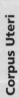

Corpus Uteri

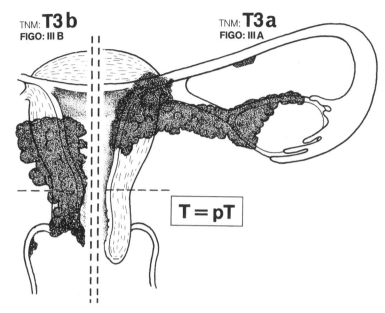

TNM: **T3 b**
FIGO: III B

TNM: **T3 a**
FIGO: III A

$T = pT$

Fig. 331

TNM: **T4**
FIGO: IVA

pT4

Fig. 332

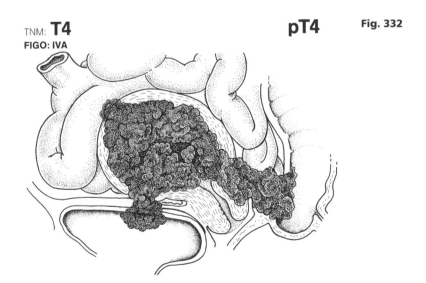

N—Regional Lymph Nodes

NX   Regional lymph nodes cannot be assessed
N0   No regional lymph node metastasis
N1   Regional lymph node metastasis (Fig. 333)

pTN Pathological Classification

The pT and pN categories correspond to the T and N categories.

pN0 Histological examination of a pelvic lymphadenectomy specimen will ordinarily include 10 or more lymph nodes.
    If the examined lymph nodes are negative, but the number ordinarily resected is not met, classify as pN0.

Fig. 333

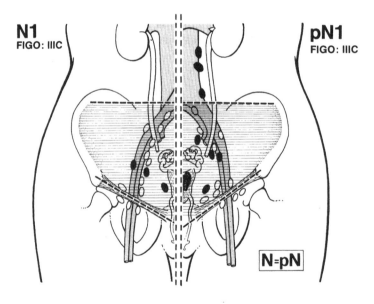

N1
FIGO: IIIC

pN1
FIGO: IIIC

N=pN

Summary

TNM	Corpus Uteri	FIGO
Tis	In situ	0
T1	Confined to corpus	I
T1a	Tumour limited to endometrium	IA
T1b	Less than half of myometrium	IB
T1c	One half or more of myometrium	IC
T2	Invades cervix	II
T2a	Endocervical glandular only	IIA
T2b	Cervical stroma	IIB
T3 and/or N1	Local or regional as specified below	III
T3a	Serosa/adnexa/positive peritoneal cytology	IIIA
T3b	Vaginal involvement	IIIB
N1	Regional lymph node metastasis	IIIC
T4	Mucosa of bladder/bowel	IVA
M1	Distant metastasis	IVB

Ovary (ICD-O C56)

The definitions of the T, N, and M categories correspond to the FIGO stages. Both systems are included for comparison.

The FIGO stages are based on clinical staging. (TNM stages are based on clinical and/or pathological classification).

Rules for Classification

The classification applies to malignant surface epithelial-stromal tumours including those of borderline malignancy or low malignant potential (WHO Classification of tumours. Pathology and Genetics. Tumours of the Breast and Female Genital Organs. Tavassoli FA, Devilee P. eds., 2003) corresponding to "common epithelial tumours" of earlier terminology. Non-epithelial ovarian cancers may also be classified using this scheme*. There should be histological confirmation of the disease and division of cases by histological type.

Note of editors:
* The FIGO classification does not cover non-epithelial ovarian cancers.

Regional Lymph Nodes (Fig. 334)

The regional lymph nodes are

(1) hypogastric (including obturator and internal iliac)
(2) common iliac
(3) external iliac
(4) lateral sacral
(5) para-aortic
(6) inguinal.

Fig. 334

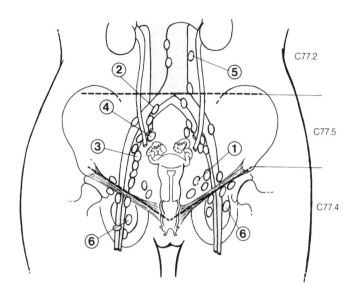

TNM Clinical Classification

T—Primary Tumour

TNM categories	FIGO stages	
TX		Primary tumour cannot be assessed
T0		No evidence of primary tumour
T1	I	Tumour limited to the ovaries
T1a	IA	Tumour limited to one ovary; capsule intact, no tumour on ovarian surface; no malignant cells in ascites or peritoneal washings (Fig. 335)
T1b	IB	Tumour limited to both ovaries; capsule intact, no tumour on ovarian surface; no malignant cells in ascites or peritoneal washings (Fig. 336)

TNM categories	FIGO stages	
T1c	IC	Tumour limited to one or both ovaries with any of the following: capsule ruptured, tumour on ovarian surface, malignant cells in ascites or peritoneal washings (Fig. 337)
T2	II	Tumour involves one or both ovaries with pelvic extension
T2a	IIA	Extension and/or implants on uterus and/or tube(s) (Fig. 338); no malignant cells in ascites or peritoneal washings
T2b	IIB	Extension to other pelvic tissues; no malignant cells in ascites or peritoneal washings (Fig. 339)
T2c	IIC	Pelvic extension (2a or 2b) with malignant cells in ascites or peritoneal washings (Fig. 340)
T3 and/or N1	III	Tumour involves one or both ovaries with microscopically confirmed peritoneal metastasis outside the pelvis and/or regional lymph node metastasis (Figs. 341–343)
T3a	IIIA	Microscopic peritoneal metastasis beyond pelvis
T3b	IIIB	Macroscopic peritoneal metastasis beyond pelvis 2.0 cm or less in greatest dimension
T3c and/or N1	IIIC	Peritoneal metastasis beyond pelvis more than 2.0 cm in greatest dimension and/or regional lymph node metastasis (Fig. 343)
M1	IV	Distant metastasis (excludes peritoneal metastasis) (Fig. 342)

Note

Liver capsule metastasis is T3/stage III, liver parenchymal metastasis M1/stage IV. Pleural effusion must have positive cytology for M1/stage IV.

Fig. 335

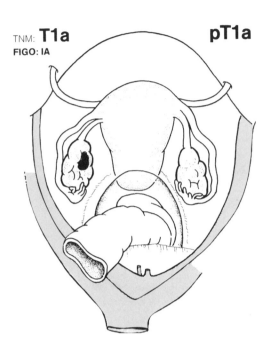

TNM: **T1a**
FIGO: IA

pT1a

Fig. 336

TNM: **T1b**
FIGO: IB

pT1b

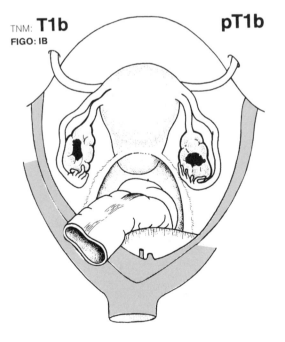

Ovary

Fig. 337

TNM: **T1c**
FIGO: IC

TNM: **T1c**
FIGO: IC

T = pT

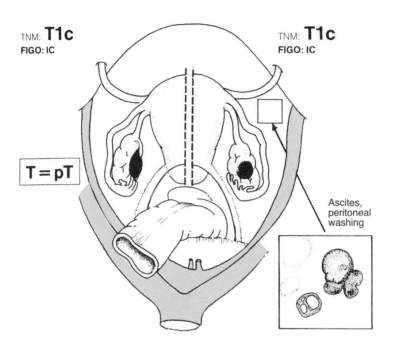

Ascites,
peritoneal
washing

Fig. 338

TNM: **T2a**
FIGO: IIA

pT2a

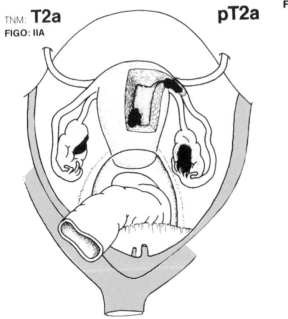

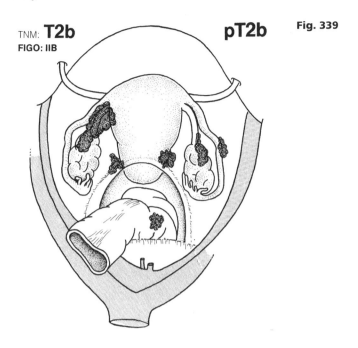

TNM: **T2b**
FIGO: IIB

pT2b

Fig. 339

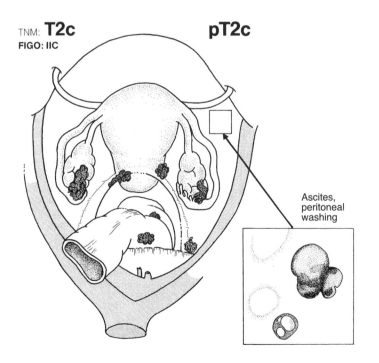

TNM: **T2c**
FIGO: IIC

pT2c

Fig. 340

Ascites, peritoneal washing

Ovary

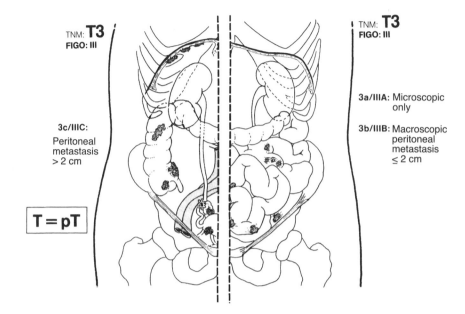

TNM: **T3**
FIGO: III

3c/IIIC:

Peritoneal
metastasis
> 2 cm

T = pT

TNM: **T3**
FIGO: III

3a/IIIA: Microscopic
only

3b/IIIB: Macroscopic
peritoneal
metastasis
≤ 2 cm

Fig. 341

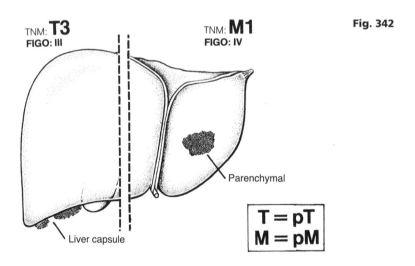

TNM: **T3**
FIGO: III

TNM: **M1**
FIGO: IV

Fig. 342

Parenchymal

Liver capsule

T = pT
M = pM

N—Regional Lymph Nodes

NX   Regional lymph nodes cannot be assessed
N0   No regional lymph node metastasis
N1   Regional lymph node metastasis (Fig. 343)

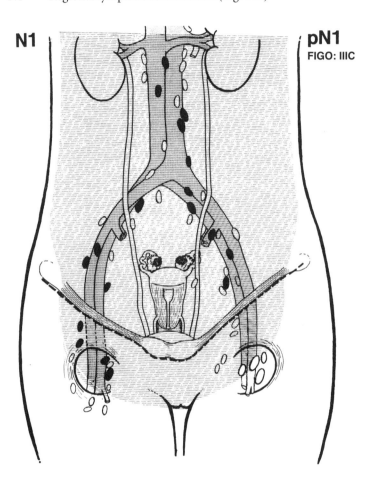

Fig. 343

N1   pN1
                                FIGO: IIIC

M—Distant Metastasis

MX   Distant metastasis cannot be assessed
M0   No distant metastasis
M1   Distant metastasis (Fig. 342, p. 288)

pTNM Pathological Classification

The pT, pN, and pM categories correspond to the T, N, and M categories.

pN0 Histological examination of a pelvic lymphadenectomy specimen will ordinarily include 10 or more lymph nodes. If the examined lymph nodes are negative, but the number ordinarily resected is not met, classify as pN0.

Summary

TNM	Ovary	FIGO
T1	Limited to the ovaries	I
T1a	One ovary, capsule intact	IA
T1b	Both ovaries, capsule intact	IB
T1c	Capsule ruptured, tumour on surface, malignant cells in ascites or peritoneal washings	IC
T2	Pelvic extension	II
T2a	Uterus, tube(s)	IIA
T2b	Other pelvic tissues	IIB
T2c	Malignant cells in ascites or peritoneal washings	IIC
T3 and/or N1	Peritoneal metastasis beyond pelvis and/or regional lymph node metastasis	III
T3a	Microscopic peritoneal metastasis	IIIA
T3b	Macroscopic peritoneal metastasis ≤ 2 cm	IIIB
T3c and/or N1	Peritoneal metastasis >2 cm and/or regional lymph node metastasis	IIIC
M1	Distant metastasis (excludes peritoneal metastasis)	IV

Fallopian Tube (ICD-O C57.0)

The definitions of the T, N, and M categories correspond to the FIGO stages. Both systems are included for comparison.

Rules for Classification

The classification applies only to carcinoma. There should be histological confirmation of the disease.

The FIGO stages are based on surgical staging. (TNM stages are based on clinical and/or pathological staging.)

Regional Lymph Nodes

The regional lymph nodes are the hypogastric (including obturator and internal iliac), common iliac, external iliac, lateral sacral, para-aortic, and inguinal nodes (see Fig. 334, p. 283)

TNM Clinical Classification

T—Primary Tumour

TNM Categories	FIGO Stages	
TX		Primary tumour cannot be assessed
T0		No evidence of primary tumour
Tis	0	Carcinoma in situ(preinvasive carcinoma)
T1	I	Tumour confined to fallopian tube(s)
T1a	IA	Tumour limited to one tube, without penetrating the serosal surface; no ascites (Fig. 344)

TNM Categories	FIGO Stages	
T1b	IB	Tumour limited to both tubes, without penetrating the serosal surface; no ascites (Fig. 345)
T1c	IC	Tumour limited to one or both tube(s) with extension onto or through the tubal serosa, or with malignant cells in ascites or peritoneal washings (Fig. 346)
T2	II	Tumour involves one or both fallopian tube(s) with pelvic extension
T2a	IIA	Extension and/or metastasis to uterus and/or ovaries (Fig. 347)
T2b	IIB	Extension to other pelvic structures (Fig. 348)
T2c	IIC	Pelvic extension (2a or 2b) with malignant cells in ascites or peritoneal washings (Fig. 349)
T3 and/or N1	III	Tumour involves one or both fallopian tube(s) with peritoneal implants outside the pelvis and/or positive regional lymph nodes
T3a	IIIA	Microscopic peritoneal metastasis outside the pelvis (Figs. 341–343, pp. 288–289)
T3b	IIIB	Macroscopic peritoneal metastasis outside the pelvis 2.0 cm or less in greatest dimension
T3c and/or N1	IIIC	Peritoneal metastasis more than 2.0 cm in greatest dimension and/or positive regional lymph nodes (Fig. 343, p. 289)
M1	IV	Distant metastasis (excludes peritoneal metastasis) (Fig. 342, p. 288)

Note:

Liver capsule metastasis is T3/stage III, liver parenchymal metastasis M1/stage IV. Pleural effusion must have positive cytology for M1/stage IV.

TNM: **T1a**
FIGO: IA

pT1a
FIGO: IA

Fig. 344

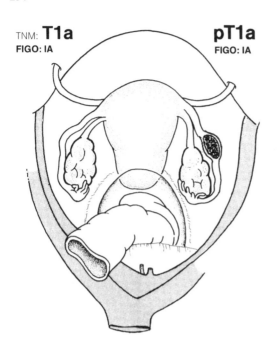

TNM: **T1b**
FIGO: IB

pT1b
FIGO: IB

Fig. 345

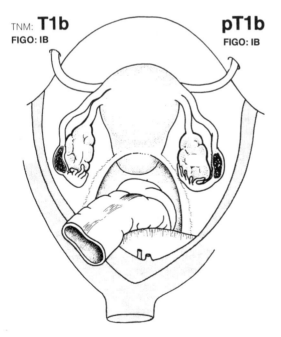

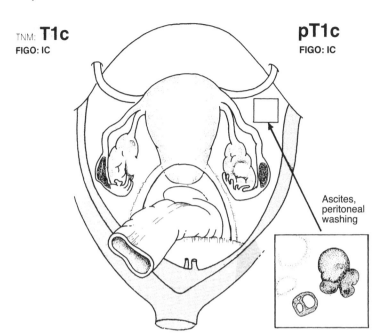

Fig. 346

TNM: **T1c**
FIGO: IC

pT1c
FIGO: IC

Ascites,
peritoneal
washing

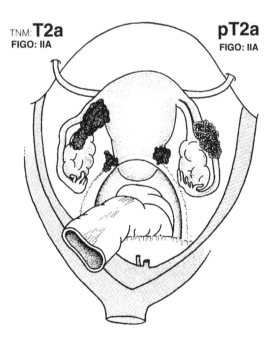

Fig. 347

TNM: **T2a**
FIGO: IIA

pT2a
FIGO: IIA

Fig. 348

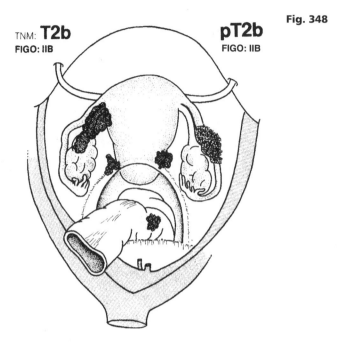

TNM: **T2b**
FIGO: IIB

pT2b
FIGO: IIB

Fig. 349

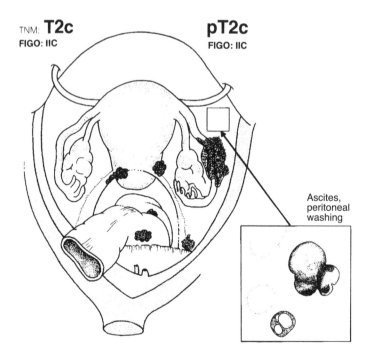

TNM: **T2c**
FIGO: IIC

pT2c
FIGO: IIC

Ascites,
peritoneal
washing

N—Regional Lymph Nodes

NX   Regional lymph nodes cannot be assessed
N0   No regional lymph node metastasis
N1   Regional lymph node metastasis (Fig. 343, p. 289)

M—Distant Metastasis

MX   Distant metastasis cannot be assessed
M0   No distant metastasis
M1   Distant metastasis (Fig. 343, p. 289)

pTNM Pathological Classification

The pT, pN, and pM categories correspond to the T, N, and M categories.

pN0 Histological examination of a pelvic lymphadenectomy specimen will ordinarily include 10 or more lymph nodes. If the examined lymph nodes are negative, but the number ordinarily resected is not met, classify as pN0.

Summary

TNM	Fallopian Tube	FIGO
T1	Limited to tube(s)	I
T1a	One tube; serosa intact	IA
T1b	Both tubes; serosa intact	IB
T1c	Serosa involved; malignant cells in ascites or peritoneal washings	IC
T2	Pelvic extension	II
T2a	Uterus and/or ovaries	IIA
T2b	Other pelvic structures	IIB
T2c	Malignant cells in ascites or peritoneal washings	IIC
T3 and/or N1	Peritoneal metastasis outside the pelvis and/or regional lymph node metastasis	III
T3a	Microscopic peritoneal metastasis	IIIA
T3b	Macroscopic peritoneal metastasis ≤ 2 cm	IIIB
T3c and/or N1	Peritoneal metastasis >2 cm and/or regional lymph node metastasis	IIIC
M1	Distant metastasis (excludes peritoneal metastasis)	IV

Fallopian Tube

Gestational Trophoblastic Tumours (ICD-O C58)

The following classification for gestational trophoblastic tumours is based on that of FIGO adopted in 1992 and updated in 2001 (Gestational trophoblastic tumours. Ngan HYS, Odicino F, Maisonneuve P, Beller U, Benedet JL, Heintz APM, Pecorelli S, Sideri M, Creasman WT. J Epidemiol Biostatist 2001;6: 175–184).

The definitions of T and M categories correspond to the FIGO stages. Both systems are included for comparison. A prognostic scoring index, which is based on factors other than the anatomic extent of the disease, is used to assign cases to high risk and low risk categories, and these categories are used in stage grouping.

Rules for Classification

The classification applies to choriocarcinoma (9100/3), invasive hydatidiform mole (9100/1), and placental site trophoblastic tumour (9104/1). Placental site tumours should be reported separately. Histological confirmation is not required if the urine human chorionic gonadotropin (hCG) level is abnormally elevated. History of prior chemotherapy for this disease should be noted.

Editor's Note
This classification should also be applied to epithelioid trophoblastic tumour (ETT).

TM Clinical Classification

T–Primary Tumour/M-Distant Metastasis

TM Categories	FIGO Stages*	
TX		Primary tumour cannot be assessed
T0		No evidence of primary tumour
T1	I	Tumour confined to uterus (Fig. 350)
T2	II	Tumour extends to other genital structures: vagina, ovary, broad ligament, fallopian tube by metastasis or direct extension (Fig. 351)
M1a	III	Metastasis to lung(s)
M1b	IV	Other distant metastasis with or without lung involvement

Note
* Stages I to IV are subdivided into A and B
  according to the prognostic score

Risk factors:		Age, antecedent pregnancy, months from index pregnancy, pretreatment serum hCG, largest tumour size including uterus, site of metastasis, number of metastasis, previous failed chemotherapy

Note
Genital metastasis (vagina, ovary, broad ligament, fallopian tube) is classified T2. Any involvement of non-genital structures, whether by direct invasion or metastasis is described using the M classification.

Prognostic score

Prognostic Factor	0	1	2	4
Age	<40	≥40		
Antecedent pregnancy	H. mole	Abortion	Term pregnancy	
Months from index pregnancy	<4	4 − <7	7 − 12	>12
Pretreatment HCG (iu/ml)	$<10^3$	$10^3 - <10^4$	$10^4 - <10^5$	$\geq10^5$
Largest tumour size including uterus	<3.0 cm	3 − <5.0 cm	≥5.0 cm	
Sites of metastasis	Lung	Spleen, kidney	Gastrointestinal tract	Liver, brain
Number of metastasis		1 − 4	5 − 8	>8
Previous failed therapy			Single drug	Two or more drugs

Risk categories:

Total prognostic score 7 or less = low risk (A)
Total score 8 or more = high risk (B)

Note

After publication of TNM 6th ed., FIGO changed their classification as follows. The FIGO stages are not subdivided into A and B; instead, they recommend adding the total prognostic score to the stage (e.g., Stage III: 4 instead of Stage IIIA); FIGO: ≤6 = low risk, ≥7 = high risk

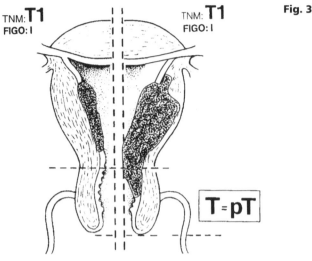

Fig. 350

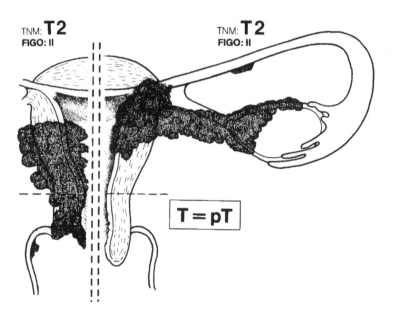

Fig. 351

pTM Pathological Classification

The pT and pM categories correspond to the T and M categories.

Summary

TM and risk	Gestational Trophoblastic Tumours	FIGO
T1	Confined to uterus	I
T2	Other genital structures	II
M1a	Metastasis to lung(s)	III
M1b	Other distant metastasis	IV
Low risk	Prognostic score 7 or less	IA–IVA
High risk	Prognostic score 8 or more	IB–IVB

Urological Tumours

Introductory Notes

The following sites are included:

- Penis
- Prostate
- Testis
- Kidney
- Renal pelvis and ureter
- Urinary bladder
- Urethra

TNM Atlas: Illustrated Guide to the TNM Classification of Malignant Tumours, Fifth Edition,
edited by Christian Wittekind, Frederick L. Greene, Robert Hutter, Martin Klimpfinger, and Leslie H. Sobin
Copyright © 2005 UICC

Penis (ICD-O C60)

Rules for Classification

The classification applies only to carcinomas. There should be histological confirmation of the disease.

Anatomical Subsites (Fig. 352)

1. Prepuce (C60.0)
2. Glans penis (C60.1)
3. Body of penis (C60.2)

Regional Lymph Nodes

The regional lymph nodes are the superficial and deep inguinal and the pelvic nodes.

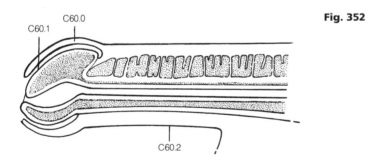

Fig. 352

TN Clinical Classification

T—Primary Tumour

TX   Primary tumour cannot be assessed
T0   No evidence of primary tumour
Tis   Carcinoma in situ
Ta   Noninvasive verrucous carcinoma (Fig. 353)

T1   Tumour invades subepithelial connective tissue (Fig. 354)
T2   Tumour invades corpus spongiosum or cavernosum (Fig. 355)
T3   Tumour invades urethra (Fig. 356) or prostate (Fig. 357)
T4   Tumour invades other adjacent structures (Figs. 358, 359)

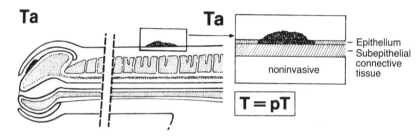

Fig. 353

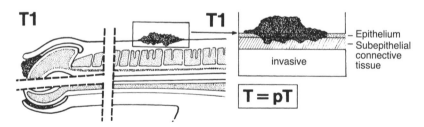

Fig. 354

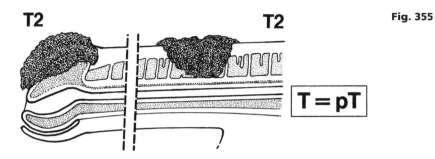

Fig. 355

T2   **T2**

$$T = pT$$

Fig. 356

T3   **T3**

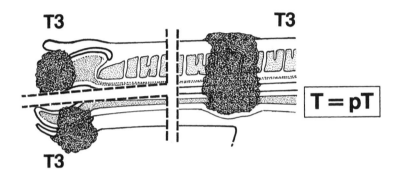

$$T = pT$$

T3

Fig. 357

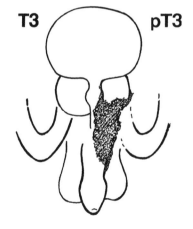

T3   **pT3**

T4   pT4

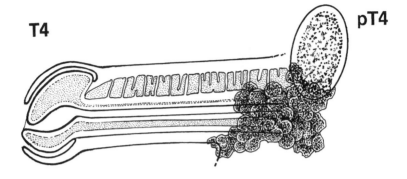

Fig. 358

T4   pT4

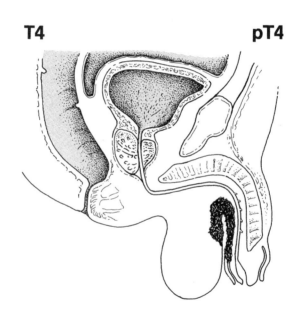

Fig. 359

N—Regional Lymph Nodes

NX   Regional lymph nodes cannot be assessed
N0   No regional lymph node metastasis
N1   Metastasis in a single superficial inguinal lymph node (Fig. 360)

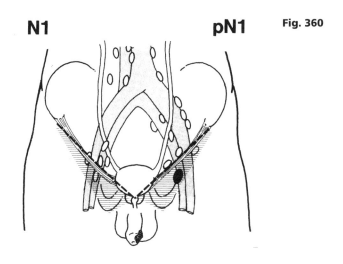

N1   **pN1**   **Fig. 360**

N2   Metastasis in multiple (Fig. 361) or bilateral superficial inguinal lymph nodes
      (Fig. 362)

Fig. 361

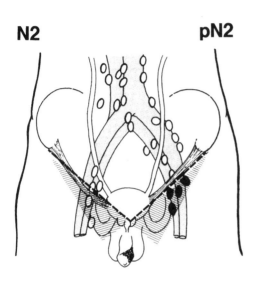

Fig. 362

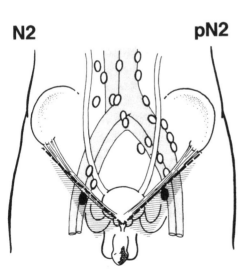

N3   Metastasis in deep inguinal (Fig. 363) or pelvic lymph node(s), unilateral
      (Fig. 364) or bilateral (Fig. 365)

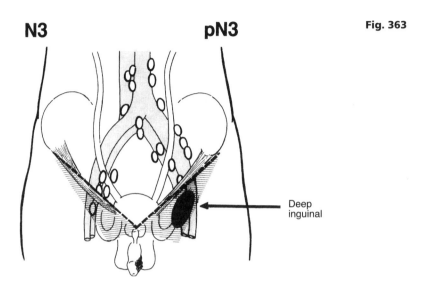

N3   **pN3**   **Fig. 363**

Deep
inguinal

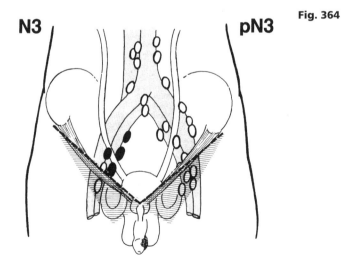

                                                  Fig. 364
N3   **pN3**

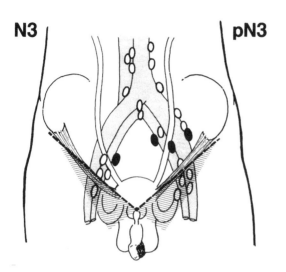

Fig. 365

N3   pN3

pTN Pathological Classification

The pT and pN categories correspond to the T and N categories.

Summary

Penis	
Tis	In situ
Ta	Noninvasive verrucous carcinoma
T1	Subepithelial connective tissue
T2	Corpus spongiosum, cavernosum
T3	Urethra, prostate
T4	Other adjacent structures
N1	One superficial inguinal
N2	Multiple or bilateral superficial inguinal
N3	Deep inguinal or pelvic

Prostate (ICD-O C61) (Figs. 366, 418, p. 356)

Rules for Classification

The classification applies only to adenocarcinomas. Transitional cell carcinoma of the prostate is classified as a urethral tumour (see p. 363 ff). There should be histological confirmation of the disease.

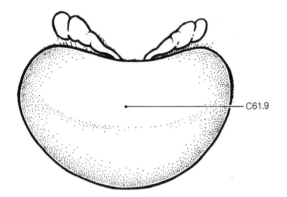

Fig. 366

C61.9

Regional Lymph Nodes (Fig. 367)

The regional lymph nodes are the nodes of the true pelvis, which essentially are the pelvic nodes below the bifurcation of the common iliac arteries. Laterality does not affect the N classification.

Fig. 367

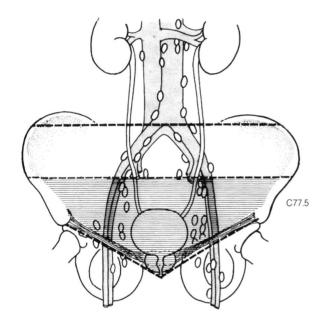

C77.5

TN Clinical Classification

T—Primary Tumour

TX   Primary tumour cannot be assessed
T0   No evidence of primary tumour

T1   Clinically inapparent tumour not palpable or visible by imaging (Fig. 368)

      T1a   Tumour incidental histological finding in 5% or less of tissue resected

      T1b   Tumour incidental histological finding in more than 5% of tissue resected

      T1c   Tumour identified by needle biopsy (e.g., because of elevated PSA)

T2   Tumour confined within the prostate[1]

      T2a   Tumour involves one half of one lobe or less (Fig. 369)

      T2b   Tumour involves more than one half of one lobe, but not both lobes (Fig. 369)

      T2c   Tumour involves both lobes (Fig. 370)

Note

[1] Tumour found in one or both lobes by needle biopsy, but not palpable or visible by imaging, is classified as T1c.

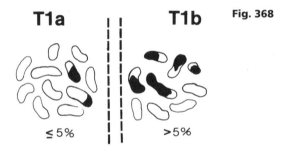

Fig. 368

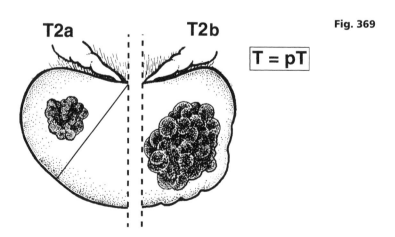

Fig. 369

$T = pT$

T3   Tumour extends through the prostatic capsule[2]
        T3a   Extracapsular extension (unilateral or bilateral) (Figs. 371, 372)
        T3b   Tumour invades seminal vesicle(s) (Fig. 373)

Note
[2] Invasion into the prostatic apex or into (but not beyond) the prostatic capsule is not classified as T3, but
    as T2.

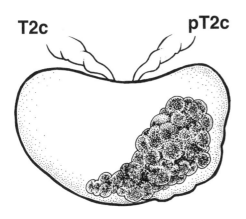

Fig. 370

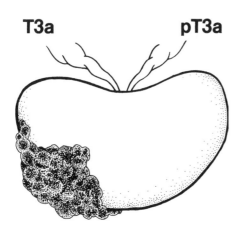

Fig. 371

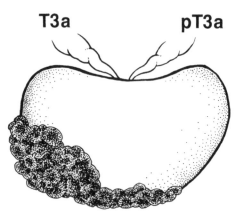

T3a   pT3a

Fig. 372

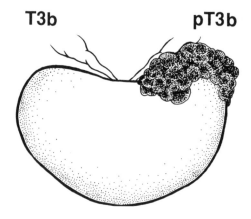

T3b   pT3b

Fig. 373

T4   Tumour is fixed or invades adjacent structures other than seminal vesicles: bladder neck, external sphincter, rectum, levator muscles, and/or pelvic wall (Figs. 374, 375)

Fig. 374

T4   **pT4**

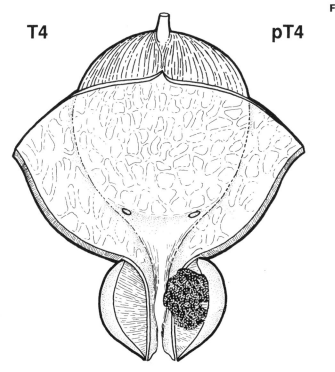

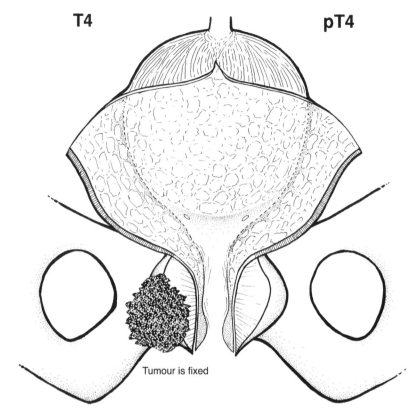

T4   **pT4**

Tumour is fixed

Fig. 375

N—Regional Lymph Nodes

NX   Regional lymph nodes cannot be assessed
N0   No regional lymph node metastasis
N1   Regional lymph node metastasis (Figs. 376, 377)

Fig. 376

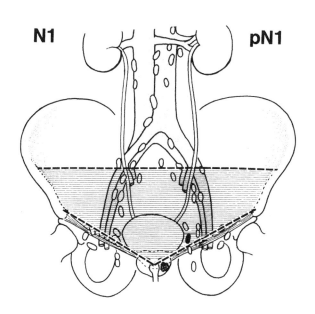

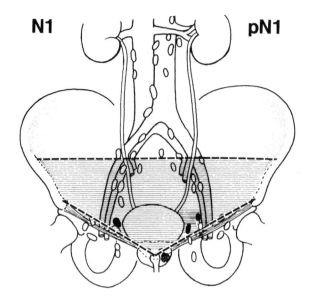

N1 **pN1**

Fig. 377

pTN Pathological Classification

The pT and pN categories correspond to the T and N categories.

However, there is no pT1 category because there is insufficient tissue to assess the highest pT category.

Note

Metastasis no larger than 0.2 cm can be designated pN1(mi).

Summary

Prostate	
T1	Not palpable or visible
T1a	≤5%
T1b	>5%
T1c	Needle biopsy
T2	Confined within prostate
T2a	≤ half of one lobe
T2b	> half of one lobe
T2c	Both lobes
T3	Through prostatic capsule
T3a	Extracapsular
T3b	Seminal vesicle(s)
T4	Fixed or invades adjacent structures: bladder neck, external sphincter, rectum, levator muscles, pelvic wall
N1	Regional lymph node(s)
M1a	Non-regional lymph node(s)
M1b	Bone(s)
M1c	Other site(s)

Testis (ICD-O C62) (Fig. 378)

Rules for Classification

The classification applies only to germ cell tumours of the testis. There should be histological confirmation of the disease and division of cases by histological type.

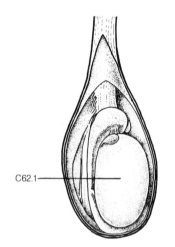

Fig. 378

C62.1

Regional Lymph Nodes (Fig. 379)

The regional lymph nodes are the abdominal para-aortic (periaortic), preaortic, interaortocaval, precaval, paracaval, retrocaval, and retroaortic nodes. Nodes along the spermatic vein should be considered regional. Laterality does not affect the N classification. The intrapelvic nodes and the inguinal nodes are considered regional after scrotal or inguinal surgery.

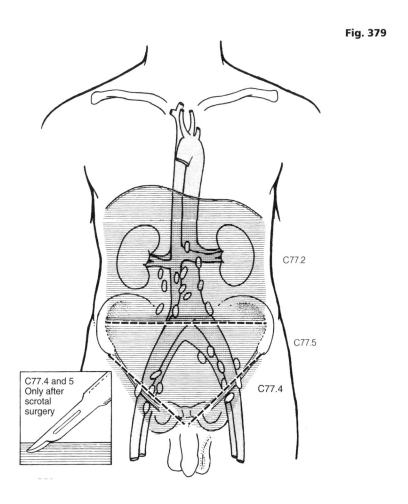

Fig. 379

C77.2

C77.5

C77.4

C77.4 and 5
Only after
scrotal
surgery

TN Clinical Classification

T—Primary Tumour

Except for pTis and pT4, where radical orchiectomy is not always necessary for classification purposes, the extent of the primary tumour is classified after radical orchiectomy; see pT. In other circumstances, TX is used if no radical orchiectomy has been performed.

N—Regional Lymph Nodes

NX   Regional lymph nodes cannot be assessed
N0   No regional lymph node metastasis
N1   Metastasis with a lymph node mass 2.0 cm or less in greatest dimension or multiple lymph nodes, none more than 2.0 cm in greatest dimension (Figs. 380–385)
N2   Metastasis with a lymph node mass more than 2.0 cm but not more than 5.0 cm in greatest dimension, or multiple lymph nodes, any one mass more than 2.0 cm but not more than 5.0 cm in greatest dimension (Figs. 386–388)
N3   Metastasis with a lymph node mass more than 5.0 cm in greatest dimension (Figs. 389–392)

N1 **pN1** Fig. 380

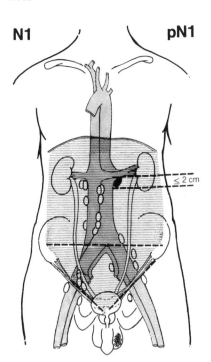

≤ 2 cm

N1 **pN1** Fig. 381

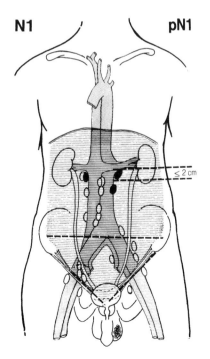

≤ 2 cm

Fig. 382

N1   pN1

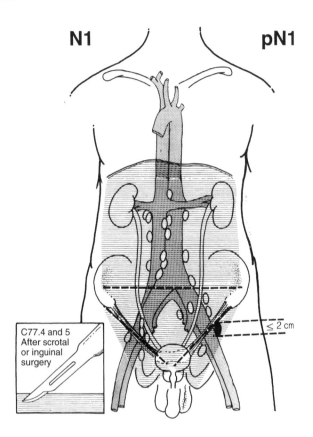

C77.4 and 5
After scrotal
or inguinal
surgery

≤ 2 cm

N1   pN1   Fig. 383

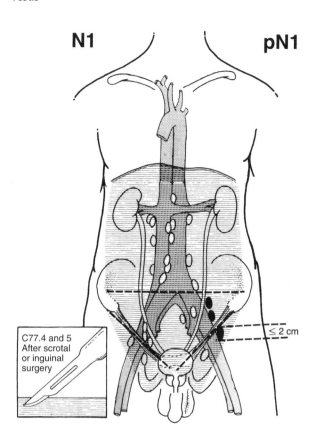

C77.4 and 5
After scrotal
or inguinal
surgery

≤ 2 cm

Testis

Fig. 384

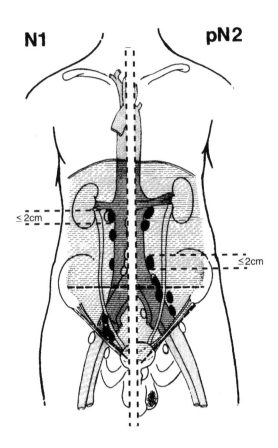

Fig. 385

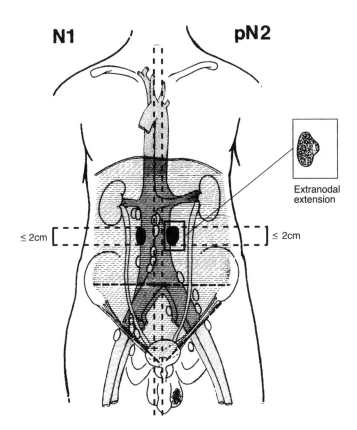

N1

pN2

Extranodal
extension

≤ 2cm

≤ 2cm

Fig. 386

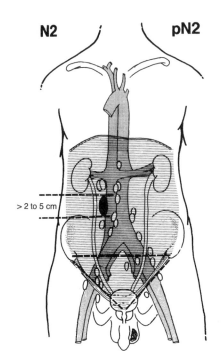

Fig. 387

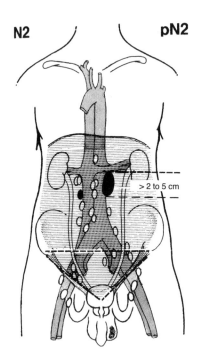

Fig. 388

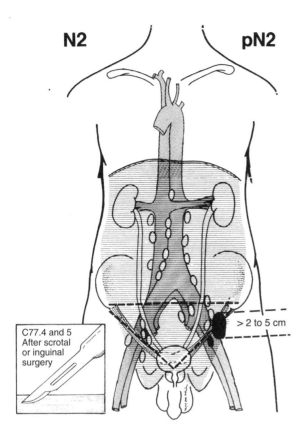

N2

pN2

> 2 to 5 cm

C77.4 and 5
After scrotal
or inguinal
surgery

Fig. 389

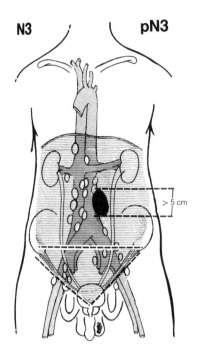

N3   pN3

> 5 cm

Fig. 390

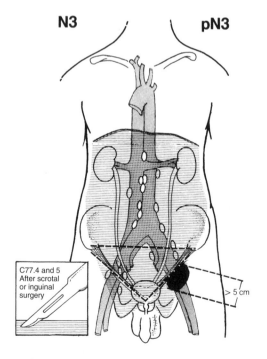

N3   pN3

C77.4 and 5
After scrotal
or inguinal
surgery

> 5 cm

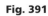

Fig. 391

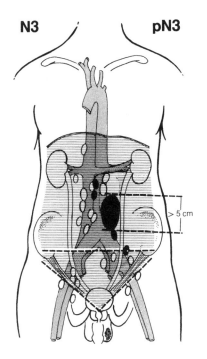

N3 pN3

> 5 cm

Fig. 392

N3 pN3

C77.4 and 5
After scrotal
or inguinal
surgery

> 5 cm

pTN Pathological Classification

pT—Primary Tumour

pTX   Primary tumour cannot be assessed (if no radical orchiectomy is performed TX is used)
pT0   No evidence of primary tumour (e.g., histologic scar in testis)
pTis Intratubular germ cell neoplasia (carcinoma in situ)

pT1   Tumour limited to testis and epididymis without vascular/lymphatic invasion; tumour may invade tunica albuginea but not tunica vaginalis (Fig. 393)
pT2   Tumour limited to testis and epididymis with vascular/lymphatic invasion (Fig. 393), or tumour extending through tunica albuginea with involvement of tunica vaginalis (Fig. 394)

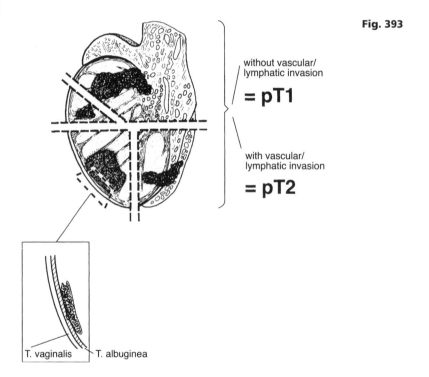

Fig. 393

without vascular/
lymphatic invasion

= pT1

with vascular/
lymphatic invasion

= pT2

T. vaginalis   T. albuginea

pT2

Fig. 394

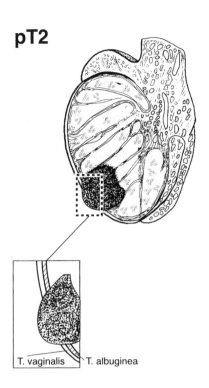

T. vaginalis   T. albuginea

pT3   Tumour invades spermatic cord with or without vascular/lymphatic invasion
       (Fig. 395)

pT4   Tumour invades scrotum with or without vascular/lymphatic invasion
       (Fig. 396)

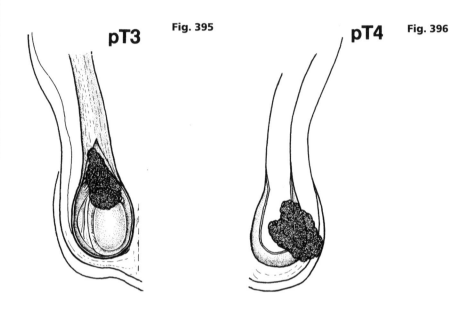

Fig. 395 pT3

Fig. 396 pT4

pN—Regional Lymph Nodes

pNX   Regional lymph nodes cannot be assessed

pN0   No regional lymph node metastasis

pN1   Metastasis with a lymph node mass 2.0 cm or less in greatest dimension and
       5 or fewer positive nodes, none more than 2.0 cm in greatest dimension
       (Figs. 380–383, pp. 327–329)

pN2   Metastasis with a lymph node mass (Figs. 384–388, pp. 330–333) more
       than 2.0 cm but not more than 5.0 cm in greatest dimension; or more than 5
       nodes positive, none more than 5.0 cm; or evidence of extranodal extension
       of tumour (Fig. 385, p. 331)

pN3   Metastasis with a lymph node mass more than 5.0 cm in greatest dimension
       (Figs. 389–392, pp. 334, 335)

Summary

Testis			
pTis	Intratubular		
pT1	Testis and epididymis, no vascular/lymphatic invasion		
pT2	Testis and epididymis with vascular/lymphatic invasion or tunica vaginalis		
pT3	Spermatic cord		
pT4	Scrotum		
N1	≤ 2 cm	pN1	≤ 2 cm and ≤ 5 nodes
N2	>2 to 5 cm	pN2	>2 to 5 cm or >5 nodes or extranodal extension
N3	>5 cm	pN3	>5 cm
M1a	Non-regional lymph nodes or lung		
M1b	Other sites		

Kidney (ICD-O C64) (Fig. 397)

Rules for Classification

The classification applies only to renal cell carcinoma. There should be histological confirmation of the disease.

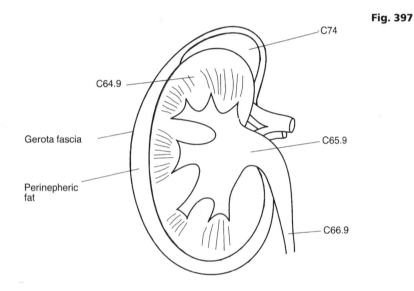

Fig. 397

Regional Lymph Nodes (Fig. 398)

The regional lymph nodes are the hilar, abdominal para-aortic (periaortic), preaortic, interaortocaval, precaval, retrocaval, and retroaortic nodes. Laterality does not affect the N classification.

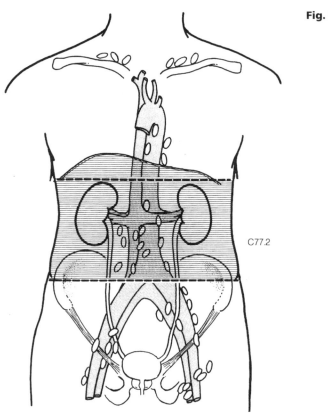

Fig. 398

C77.2

TN Clinical Classification

T—Primary Tumour (Fig. 420)

TX   Primary tumour cannot be assessed
T0   No evidence of primary tumour

T1   Tumour 7.0 cm or less in greatest dimension, limited to the kidney
      T1a   Tumour 4.0 cm or less in greatest dimension, limited to the kidney
           (Fig. 399)
      T1b   Tumour more than 4.0 cm but not more than 7.0 cm in greatest
           dimension; limited to the kidney (Fig. 400)

T1a   **pT1a**   Fig. 399

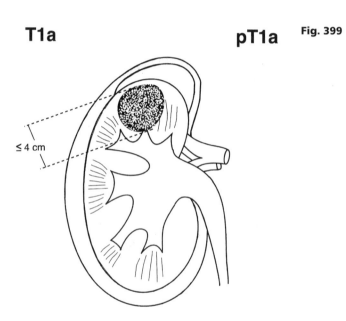

≤ 4 cm

Kidney

Fig. 400

T1b   pT1b

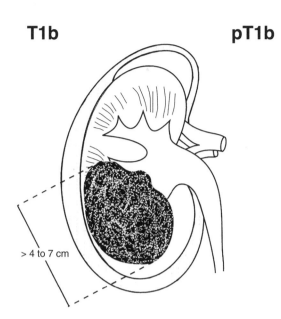

> 4 to 7 cm

T2   Tumour more than 7.0 cm in greatest dimension, limited to the kidney
(Fig. 401)

T3   Tumour extends into major veins or directly invades adrenal gland or
perinephric tissues but not beyond Gerota fascia

        T3a   Tumour directly invades adrenal gland or perinephric tissues[1] but
not beyond Gerota fascia (Fig. 402)

        T3b   Tumour grossly extends into renal vein(s)[2] or vena cava below
diaphragm (Fig. 403)

        T3c   Tumour grossly extends into vena cava above diaphragm (Fig. 404)

Notes

[1] Includes renal sinus (peripelvic) fat

[2] Includes segmental (muscle-containing) branches

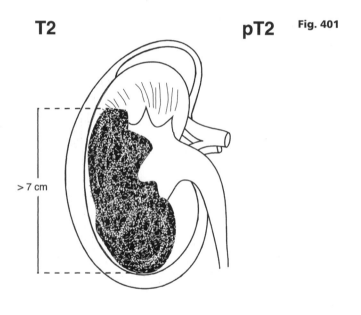

T2   pT2   **Fig. 401**

> 7 cm

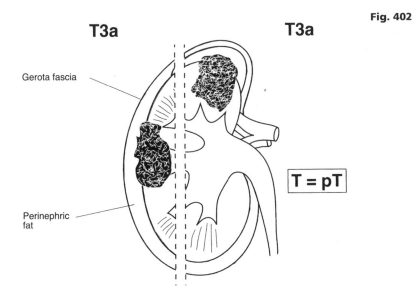

T3a

T3a

Gerota fascia

Perinephric fat

$$T = pT$$

Fig. 402

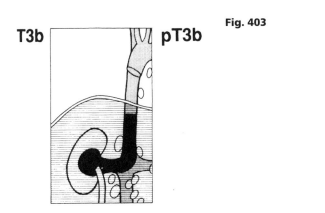

T3b **pT3b**

Fig. 403

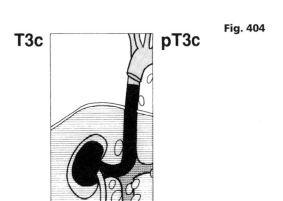

T3c **pT3c**

Fig. 404

T4   Tumour directly invades beyond Gerota fascia (Fig. 405)

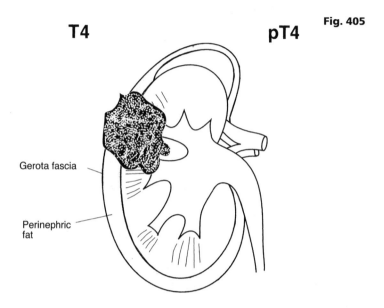

T4   **pT4**   Fig. 405

Gerota fascia

Perinephric
fat

N—Regional Lymph Nodes

NX   Regional lymph nodes cannot be assessed
N0   No regional lymph node metastasis
N1   Metastasis in a single regional lymph node (Fig. 406)
N2   Metastasis in more than one regional lymph node (Fig. 407)

Fig. 406

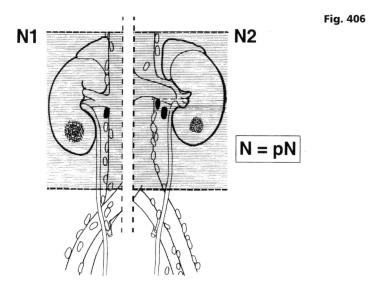

N1   N2

$$N = pN$$

Fig. 407

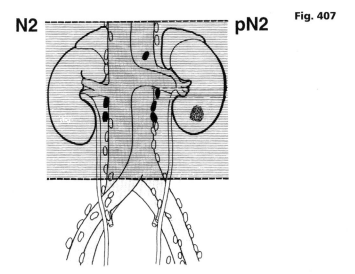

N2   pN2

pTN Pathological Classification

The pT and pN categories correspond to the T and N categories.

Summary

Kidney	
T1	≤7 cm; limited to the kidney
T1a	≤4 cm
T1b	>4 cm
T2	>7 cm; limited to the kidney
T3	Adrenal or perinephric invasion; major veins
T3a	Adrenal or perinephric invasion
T3b	Renal vein(s), vena cava below diaphragm
T3c	Vena cava above diaphragm
T4	Beyond Gerota fascia
N1	Single
N2	More than one

Renal Pelvis and Ureter (ICD-O C65, C66)

Rules for Classification

The classification applies only to carcinomas. Papilloma is excluded. There should be histological or cytological confirmation of the disease.

Anatomical Sites (Fig. 397, p. 340)

1. Renal pelvis (C65.9)
2. Ureter (C66.9)

Regional Lymph Nodes (Fig. 399, p. 342)

The regional lymph nodes are the hilar, abdominal para-aortic (periaortic), preaortic, interaortocaval, retrocaval and retroaortic nodes, and, for ureter, intrapelvic nodes. Laterality does not affect the N categories.

TN Clinical Classification

T—Primary Tumour

TX   Primary tumour cannot be assessed
T0   No evidence of primary tumour
Ta   Noninvasive papillary carcinoma (Fig. 408)
Tis   Carcinoma in situ

T1   Tumour invades subepithelial connective tissue (Fig. 408)
T2   Tumour invades muscularis (Fig. 408)
T3   *(Renal pelvis)* Tumour invades beyond muscularis into peripelvic fat or renal parenchyma (Fig. 409)
       (Ureter) Tumour invades beyond muscularis into periureteric fat (Fig. 409)

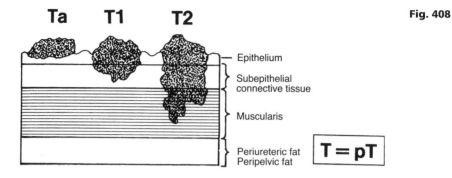

Fig. 408

Epithelium

Subepithelial
connective tissue

Muscularis

Periureteric fat
Peripelvic fat

$$T = pT$$

Fig. 409

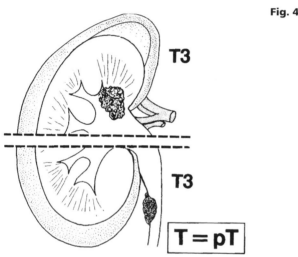

$$T = pT$$

T4   Tumour invades adjacent organs (Figs. 410, 411) or through the kidney into perinephric fat (Fig. 412)

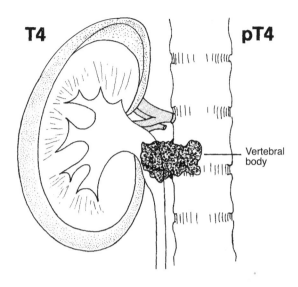

Fig. 410

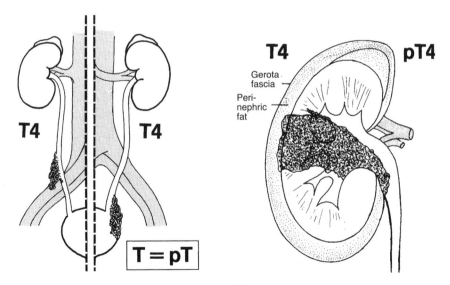

Fig. 411   **Fig. 412**

N—Regional Lymph Nodes

NX   Regional lymph nodes cannot be assessed
N0   No regional lymph node metastasis
N1   Metastasis in a single lymph node 2.0 cm or less in greatest dimension
     (Fig. 413)
N2   Metastasis in a single lymph node more than 2.0 cm but not more than
     5.0 cm in greatest dimension (Fig. 414), or multiple lymph nodes, none more
     than 5.0 cm in greatest dimension (Fig. 415)
N3   Metastasis in a lymph node more than 5.0 cm in greatest dimension
     (Figs. 416, 417)

N1 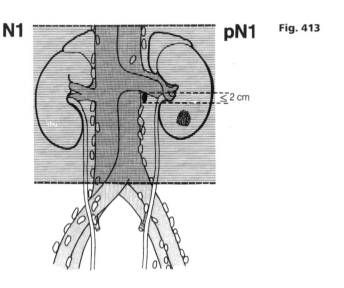 **pN1**   Fig. 413

≤ 2 cm

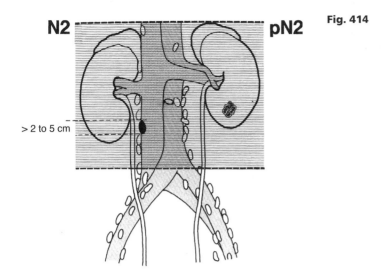

N2 pN2 Fig. 414

> 2 to 5 cm

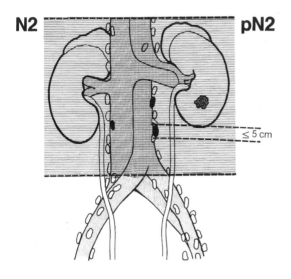

N2 pN2 Fig. 415

≤ 5 cm

Fig. 416

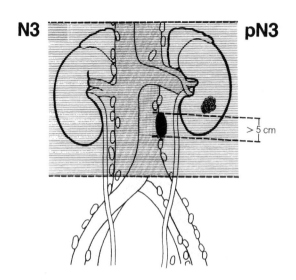

Fig. 417

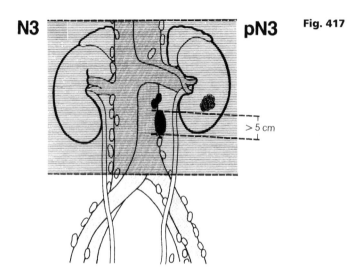

pTN Pathological Classification

The pT and pN categories correspond to the T and N categories.

Summary

Renal Pelvis, Ureter	
Ta	Noninvasive papillary
Tis	In situ
T1	Subepithelial connective tissue
T2	Muscularis
T3	Beyond muscularis
T4	Adjacent organs, perinephric fat
N1	Single ≤2 cm
N2	Single >2 to 5 cm, multiple ≤5 cm
N3	>5 cm

Urinary Bladder (ICD-O C67)

Rules for Classification

The classification applies only to carcinomas. Papilloma is excluded. There should be histological or cytological confirmation of the disease.

Anatomical Subsites (Fig. 418)

1. Trigone (C67.0)
2. Dome (C67.1)
3. Lateral wall (C67.2)
4. Anterior wall (C67.3)
5. Posterior wall (C67.4)
6. Bladder neck (C67.5)
7. Ureteric orifice (C67.6)
8. Urachus (C67.7)

Fig. 418

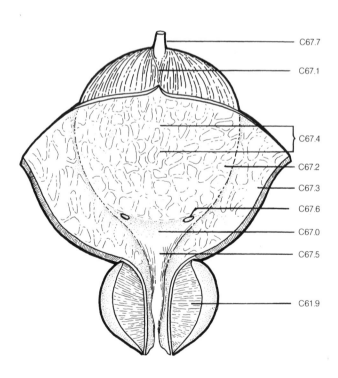

356

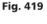

Fig. 419

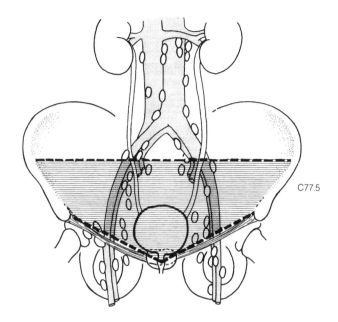

C77.5

Regional Lymph Nodes (Fig. 419)

The regional lymph nodes are the nodes of the true pelvis, which essentially are the pelvic nodes below the bifurcation of the common iliac arteries. Laterality does not affect the N classification.

TN Clinical Classification

T—Primary Tumour (Fig. 420)

The suffix (m) should be added to the appropriate T category to indicate multiple tumours. The suffix (is) may be added to any T to indicate presence of associated carcinoma in situ.

TX	Primary tumour cannot be assessed
T0	No evidence of primary tumour
Ta	Noninvasive papillary carcinoma
Tis	Carcinoma in situ: "flat tumour"

T1   Tumour invades subepithelial connective tissue
T2   Tumour invades muscle
         T2a   Tumour invades superficial muscle (inner half)
         T2b   Tumour invades deep muscle (outer half)
T3   Tumour invades perivesical tissue:
         T3a   Microscopically
         T3b   Macroscopically (extravesical mass)
T4   Tumour invades any of the following: prostate, uterus, vagina, pelvic wall, abdominal wall
         T4a   Tumour invades prostate or uterus or vagina
         T4b   Tumour invades pelvic wall or abdominal wall

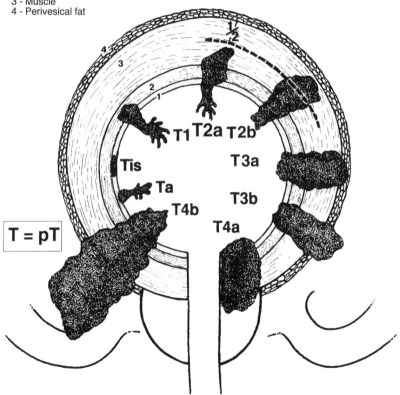

1 - Epithelium
2 - Subepithelial connective tissue
3 - Muscle
4 - Perivesical fat

Fig. 420

N—Regional Lymph Nodes

NX Regional lymph nodes cannot be assessed
N0 No regional lymph node metastasis
N1 Metastasis in a single lymph node 2.0 cm or less in greatest dimension (Fig. 421)
N2 Metastasis in a single lymph node more than 2.0 cm but not more than 5.0 cm in greatest dimension (Fig. 422), or multiple lymph nodes, none more than 5.0 cm in greatest dimension (Fig. 423)
N3 Metastasis in a lymph node more than 5 cm in greatest dimension (Figs. 424, 425)

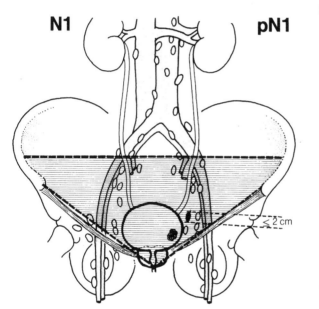

Fig. 421

N1　pN1

≤ 2 cm

Fig. 422

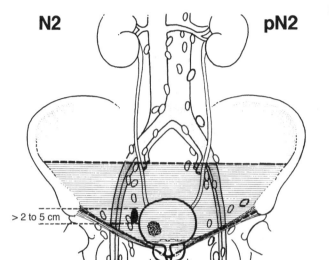

N2   pN2

> 2 to 5 cm

Fig. 423

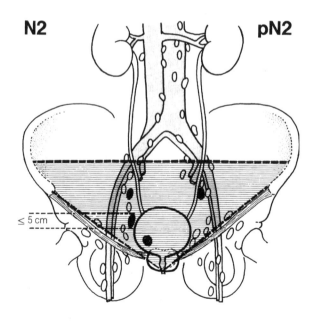

N2   pN2

≤ 5 cm

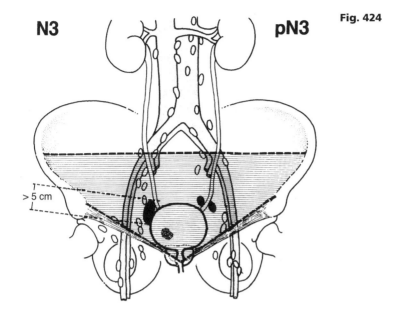

Fig. 424

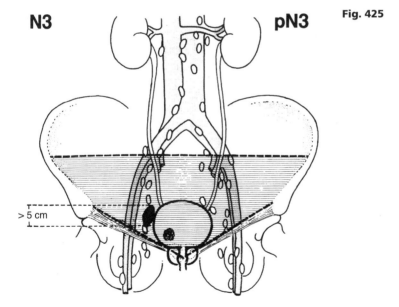

Fig. 425

pTN Pathological Classification

The pT and pN categories correspond to the T and N categories.

Summary

Urinary Bladder	
Ta	Noninvasive papillary
Tis	In situ: "flat tumour"
T1	Subepithelial connective tissue
T2	Muscularis
T2a	Inner half
T2b	Outer half
T3	Beyond muscularis
T3a	Microscopically
T3b	Extravesical mass
T4a	Prostate, uterus, vagina
T4b	Pelvic wall, abdominal wall
N1	Single ≤2 cm
N2	Single >2 to 5 cm, multiple ≤5 cm
N3	>5 cm

Urethra

Rules for Classification

The classification applies to carcinomas of the urethra (ICD-O C68.0) and transitional cell carcinomas of the prostate (ICD-O C61.9) and prostatic urethra. There should be histological or cytological confirmation of the disease.

Regional Lymph Nodes (Fig. 379, p. 325)

The regional lymph nodes are the inguinal and the pelvic nodes. Laterality does not affect the N classification.

TN Clinical Classification

T—Primary Tumour

TX   Primary tumour cannot be assessed
T0   No evidence of primary tumour

Urethra (male and female)

Ta   Noninvasive papillary, polypoid, or verrucous carcinoma (Figs. 426, 427)
Tis   Carcinoma in situ

T1   Tumour invades subepithelial connective tissue (Figs. 426, 428)
T2   Tumour invades any of the following: corpus spongiosum, prostate, peri-urethral muscle (Figs. 426, 429, 430)
T3   Tumour invades any of the following: corpus cavernosum, beyond prostatic capsule, anterior vagina, bladder neck (Figs. 431–433)
T4   Tumour invades other adjacent organs (Fig. 434)

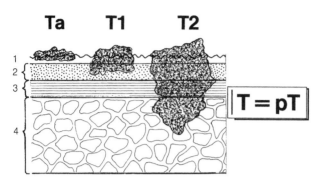

Fig. 426. *1* Epithelium, *2* subepithelial connective tissue, *3* urethral muscle, *4* urogenital diaphragm

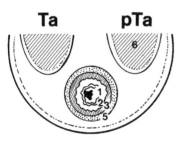

Fig. 427. *1* Epithelium, *2* subepithelial connective tissue, *3* urethral muscle, *5* corpus spongiosum, *6* corpus cavernosum

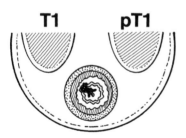

Fig. 428

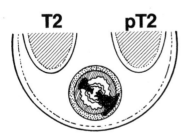

Fig. 429

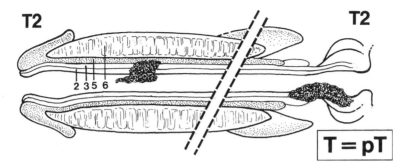

Fig. 430. *2,3,5,6: See Fig. 427*

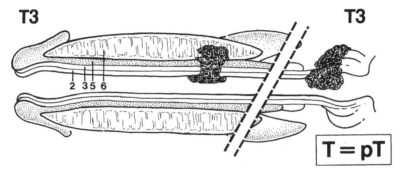

Fig. 431. *2,3,5,6: See Fig. 427*

Fig. 432

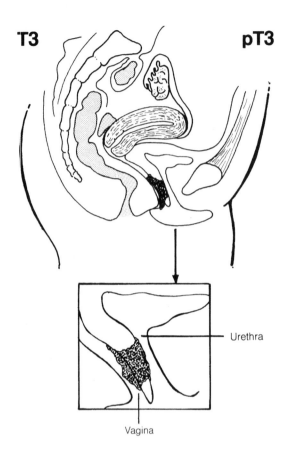

T3

pT3

Urethra

Vagina

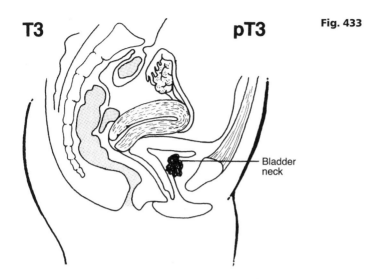

T3   **pT3**   Fig. 433

Bladder
neck

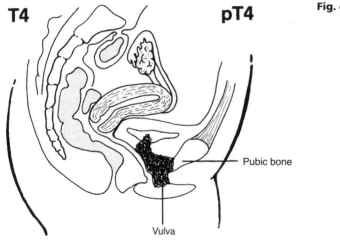

T4   **pT4**   Fig. 434

Pubic bone

Vulva

Transitional cell carcinoma of prostate (prostatic urethra)

Tis pu   Carcinoma in situ, involvement of prostatic urethra (Fig. 435)
Tis pd   Carcinoma in situ, involvement of prostatic ducts (Fig. 436)

T1   Tumour invades subepithelial connective tissue (Figs. 435, 436)
T2   Tumour invades any of the following: prostatic stroma, corpus spongiosum, periurethral muscle (Figs. 436, 437)
T3   Tumour invades any of the following: corpus cavernosum, beyond prostatic capsule, bladder neck (extraprostatic extension) (Fig. 438)
T4   Tumour invades other adjacent organs (invasion of the bladder) (Fig. 439)

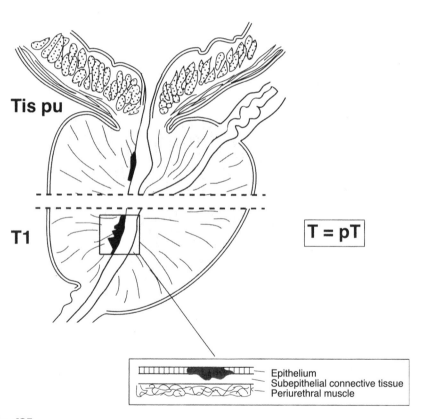

Fig. 435

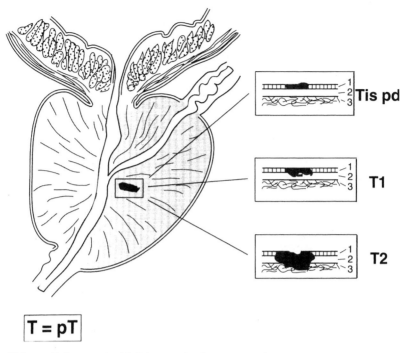

$$\boxed{T = pT}$$

Fig. 436. *1* Epithelium, *2* subepithelial connective tissue, *3* prostatic stroma

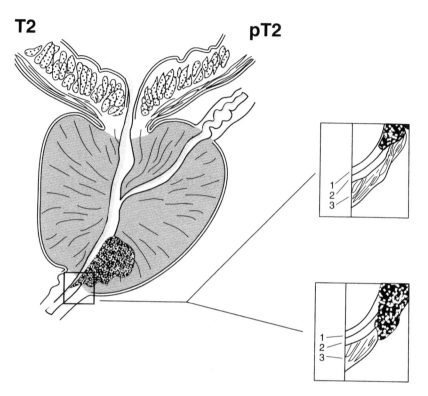

Fig. 437. *1* Urethral epithelium and subepithelial connective tissue, *2* periurethral muscle, *3* corpus spongiosum

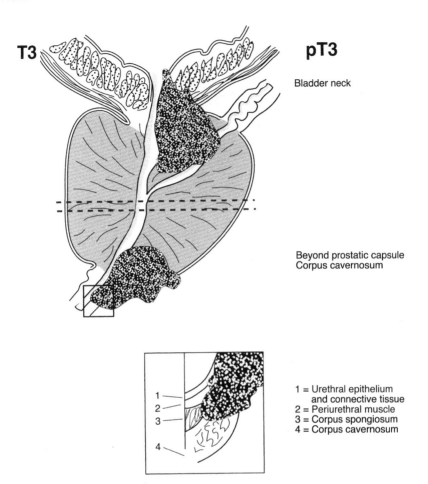

T3

pT3

Bladder neck

Beyond prostatic capsule
Corpus cavernosum

1 = Urethral epithelium
    and connective tissue
2 = Periurethral muscle
3 = Corpus spongiosum
4 = Corpus cavernosum

Fig. 438

T4

pT4

Fig. 439

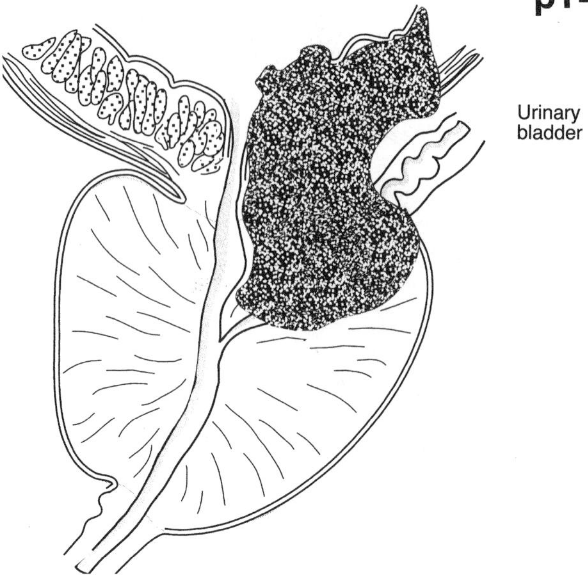

Urinary
bladder

N—Regional Lymph Nodes

NX   Regional lymph nodes cannot be assessed
N0   No regional lymph node metastasis
N1   Metastasis in a single lymph node 2.0 cm or less in greatest dimension
      (Fig. 440)

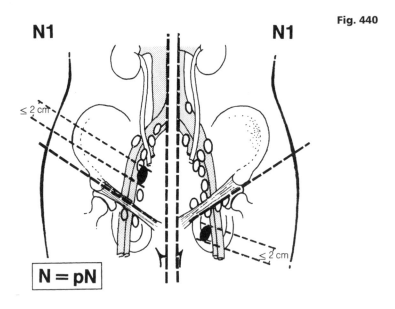

Fig. 440

N1   **N1**

N2   Metastasis in a single lymph node more than 2.0 cm in greatest dimension (Fig. 441), or multiple lymph nodes (Fig. 442)

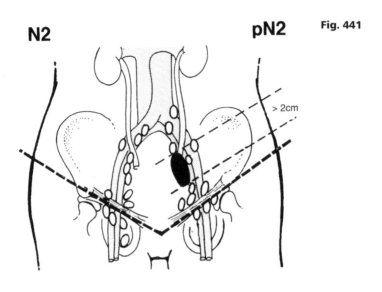

N2   **pN2**   **Fig. 441**

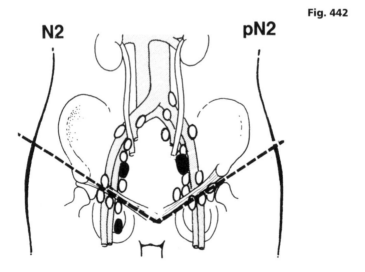

Fig. 442

N2   **pN2**

pTN Pathological Classification

The pT and pN categories correspond to the T and N categories.

Summary

Urethra	
Ta	Noninvasive papillary, polypoid, or verrucous
Tis	In situ
T1	Subepithelial connective tissue
T2	Corpus spongiosum, prostate, periurethral muscle
T3	Corpus cavernosum, beyond prostatic capsule, anterior vagina, bladder neck
T4	Other adjacent organs
Transitional Cell Carcinoma of Prostate (Prostatic Urethra)	
Tis pu	In situ, prostatic urethra
Tis pd	In situ, prostatic ducts
T1	Subepithelial connective tissue
T2	Prostatic stroma, corpus spongiosum, periurethral muscle
T3	Corpus cavernosum, beyond prostatic capsule, bladder neck (extraprostatic extension)
T4	Other adjacent organs (bladder)
N1	Single ≤2 cm
N2	>2 cm or multiple

Ophthalmic Tumours

Introductory Notes

Tumours of the eye and its adnexa are a disparate group including carcinoma, melanoma, sarcomas, and retinoblastoma. For clinical convenience they are classified in one section.

- Eyelid (eyelid melanoma is classified with skin tumours)
- Conjunctiva
- Uvea
- Retina
- Orbit
- Lacrimal gland

Regional Lymph Nodes (Fig. 443)

The regional lymph nodes are the preauricular (1), submandibular (2) and cervical (3) lymph nodes.

Fig. 443

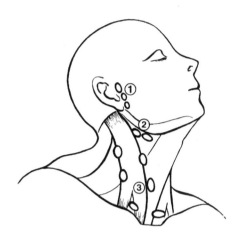

The definitions of N categories for ophthalmic tumours are:

N—Regional Lymph Nodes

NX   Regional lymph nodes cannot be assessed
N0   No regional lymph node metastasis
N1   Regional lymph node metastasis

Carcinoma of Eyelid (ICD-O C44.1)

Rules of Classification

There should be histological confirmation of the disease and division of cases by histological type, e.g., basal cell, squamous cell, sebaceous carcinoma.

T Clinical Classification

T—Primary Tumour

TX   Primary tumour cannot be assessed
T0   No evidence of primary tumour
Tis   Carcinoma in situ

T1   Tumour of any size, not invading the tarsal plate; or at eyelid margin, 5.0 mm or less in greatest dimension (Fig. 444a, b)

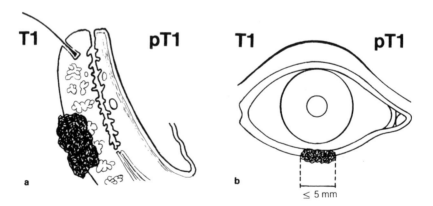

Fig. 444a, b

T2   Tumour invades tarsal plate; or at eyelid margin, more than 5.0 mm but not more than 10.0 mm in greatest dimension (Fig. 445a, b)

T3   Tumour involves full eyelid thickness; or at eyelid margin, more than 10.0 mm in greatest dimension (Fig. 446a, b)

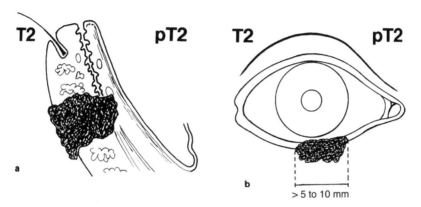

Fig. 445a, b

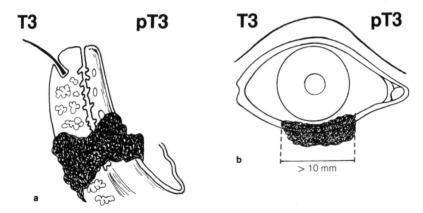

Fig. 446a, b

T4   Tumour invades adjacent structures, which include bulbar conjunctiva, sclera/globe, soft tissues of the orbit, perineural invasion, bone/periosteum of the orbit, nasal cavity/paranasal sinuses, and central nervous system (Fig. 447a, b)

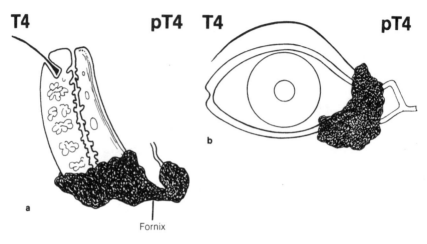

Fig. 447a, b

pT Pathological Classification

The pT categories correspond to the T categories.

Summary

Eyelid Carcinoma	
T1	Not in tarsal plate Lid margin: ≤5 mm
T2	In tarsal plate Lid margin: >5 to 10 mm
T3	Full thickness Lid margin: >10 mm
T4	Adjacent structures
N1	Regional

Carcinoma of Conjunctiva (ICD-O C 69.0)

Rules for Classification

There should be histological confirmation of the disease and division of cases by histological type, e.g., mucoepidermoid and squamous cell carcinoma.

T Clinical Classification

T—Primary Tumour

TX   Primary tumour cannot be assessed
T0   No evidence of primary tumour
Tis   Carcinoma in situ

T1   Tumour 5.0 mm or less in greatest dimension (Fig. 448)
T2   Tumour more than 5.0 mm in greatest dimension, without invasion of adjacent structures (Fig. 449)

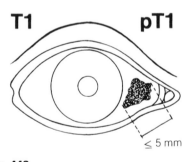

Fig. 448

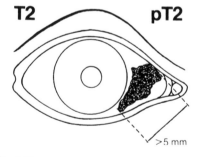

Fig. 449

T3   Tumour invades adjacent structures, excluding the orbit (Fig. 450)
T4   Tumour invades the orbit
     T4a   Tumour invades orbital soft tissues (Fig. 451a, b)

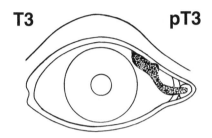

Fig. 450

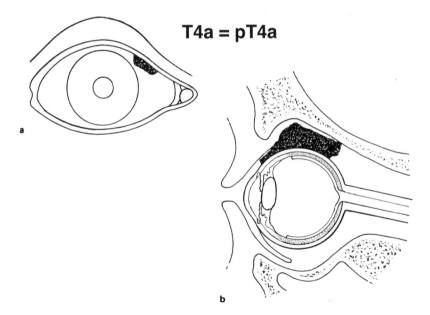

Fig. 451a, b

T4b   Tumour invades bone (Fig. 452a, b)
T4c   Tumour invades paranasal sinuses (Fig. 453a, b)

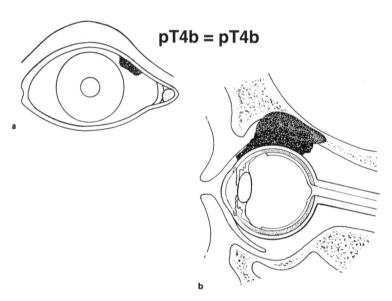

pT4b = pT4b

Fig. 452a, b

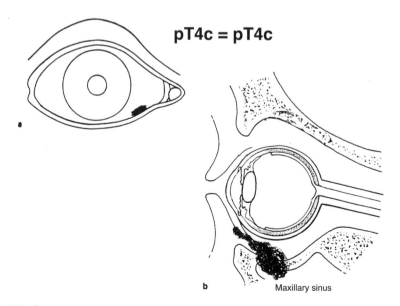

pT4c = pT4c

Maxillary sinus

Fig. 453a, b

T4d   Tumour invades brain (Fig. 454a, b)

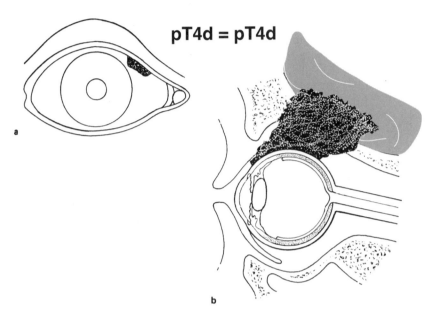

Fig. 454a, b

pT Pathological Classification

The pT categories correspond to the T categories.

Summary

Conjunctiva Carcinoma	
T1	≤5 mm
T2	>5 mm without invasion of adjacent structures
T3	Adjacent structures excluding orbit
T4	Orbit and beyond
N1	Regional

Malignant Melanoma of Conjunctiva (ICD-O C69.0)

Rules for Classification

The classification applies only to malignant melanoma. There should be histological confirmation of the disease.

T Clinical Classification

T—Primary Tumour

TX Primary tumour cannot be assessed
T0 No evidence of primary tumour

T1 Tumour(s) of bulbar conjunctiva (Figs. 455, 456)

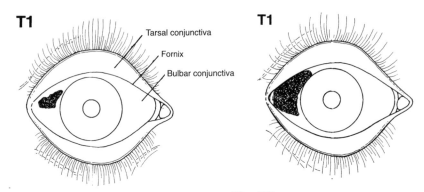

Fig. 455

Fig. 456

T2   Tumour(s) of bulbar conjunctiva with corneal extension (Fig. 457)
T3   Tumour(s) extends into conjunctival fornix, palpebral conjunctiva, or
      caruncle (Fig. 458)

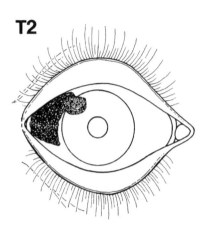

T2   **Fig. 457**

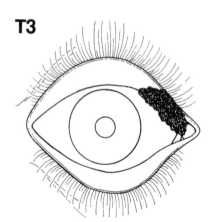

T3   **Fig. 458**

T4 Tumour invades eyelid (Fig. 459), globe, orbit, sinuses, or central nervous system

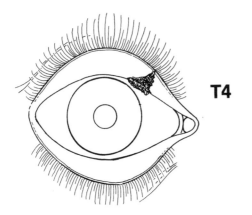

Fig. 459

T4

pT Pathological Classification

pT—Primary Tumour

pTX   Primary tumour cannot be assessed
pT0   No evidence of primary tumour

pT1   Tumour(s) of bulbar conjunctiva confined to the epithelium
pT2   Tumour(s) of bulbar conjunctiva occupying not more than 0.8 mm in thickness with invasion of the substantia propria (Fig. 460)

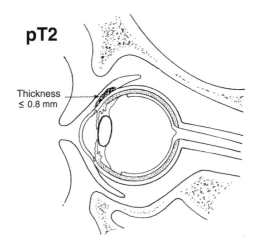

Fig. 460

pT2

Thickness ≤ 0.8 mm

pT3 Tumour(s) of bulbar conjunctiva more than 0.8 mm in thickness with invasion of the substantia propria or tumour(s) involving the palpebral or caruncular conjunctiva (Fig. 461)

pT4 Tumour(s) invade(s) eyelid, globe, orbit, sinuses, or central nervous system (Fig. 462)

pT3

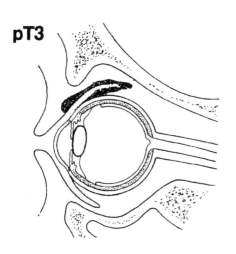

Fig. 461

pT4

Fig. 462

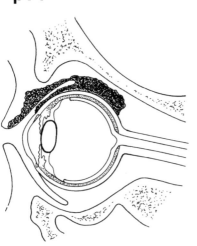

Summary

Malignant Melanoma of Conjunctiva			
T1	Bulbar conjunctiva	pT1	T1 confined to epithelium
T2	Bulbar conjunctiva with corneal extension	pT2	Bulbar conjunctiva ≤0.8 mm thick, invades substantia propria
T3	Fornix, palpebral conjunctiva, caruncle	pT3	pT2 >0.8 mm thick or involves palpebral or caruncular conjunctiva
T4	Eyelid, globe, orbit, sinuses, CNS	pT4	T4
N1	Regional	pN1	Regional

Malignant Melanoma of Uvea

(ICD-O C69.3,4)

Rules for Classification

There should be histological confirmation of the disease.

Anatomical Sites

1. Iris (C69.4)
2. Ciliary body (C69.4)
3. Choroid (C69.3)

T: Clinical Classification

T—Primary Tumour

TX	Primary tumour cannot be assessed
T0	No evidence of primary tumour

Iris

T1	Tumour limited to the iris	
	T1a	not more than 3 clock hours in size (Fig. 463a, b)
	T1b	more than 3 clock hours in size (Fig. 464a, b)
	T1c	with melanomalytic glaucoma

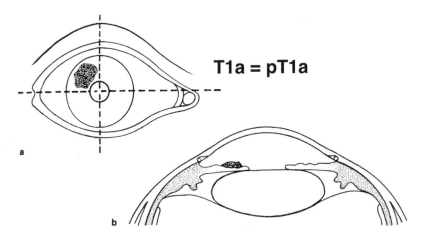

Fig. 463a, b

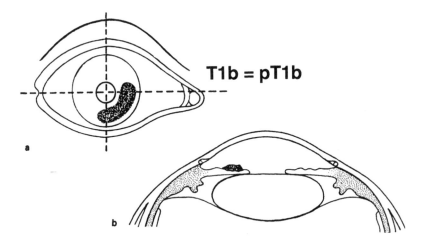

Fig. 464a, b

T2   Tumour confluent with or extending into the ciliary body or choroid
      (Fig. 465a, b)
      T2a   with melanomalytic glaucoma
T3   Tumour with scleral extension (Fig. 466a, b)
      T3a   Tumour with scleral extension *and* melanomalytic glaucoma

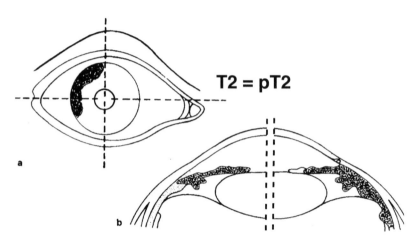

Fig. 465a, b

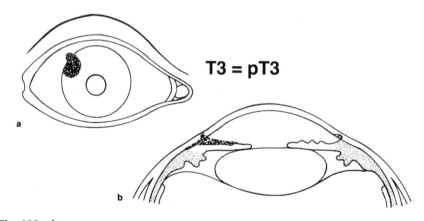

Fig. 466a, b

T4 Tumour with extraocular extension (Fig. 467a, b)

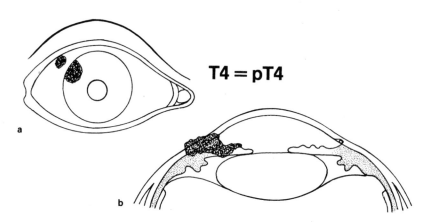

T4 = pT4

Fig. 467a, b

Ciliary Body and Choroid

T1   Tumour 10 mm or less in greatest diameter and 2.5 mm or less in greatest height (thickness) (Figs. 468, 469a, b)

    T1a   Without extraocular extension
    T1b   With microscopic extraocular extension
    T1c   With macroscopic extraocular extension

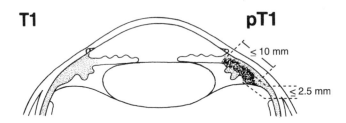

Fig. 468

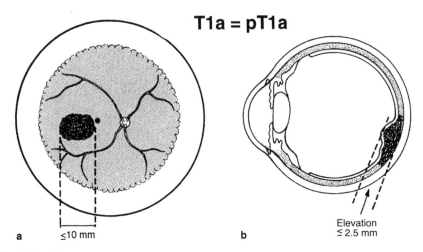

a   ≤10 mm   b   Elevation ≤ 2.5 mm

Fig. 469a, b

T2 Tumour greater than 10 mm and not more than 16 mm in greatest diameter and more than 2.5 mm and 10 mm in greatest height (Figs. 470, 471a, b)

T2a without extraocular extension
T2b with microscopic extraocular extension
T2c with macroscopic extraocular extension

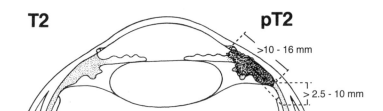

Fig. 470

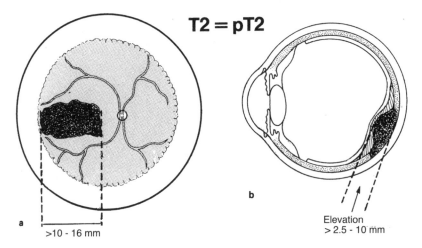

Fig. 471a, b

T3   Tumour more than 16 mm in greatest diameter and/or greater than 10 mm
       in greatest height, *without* extraocular extension (Figs. 472, 473a, b)

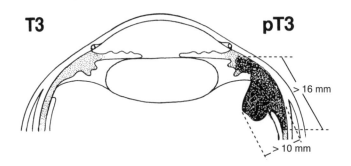

Fig. 472

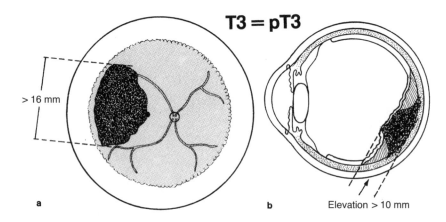

a   b   Elevation > 10 mm

Fig. 473a, b

T4   Tumour more than 16 mm in greatest diameter and/or greater than 10 mm in greatest height *with* extraocular extension (Figs. 474, 475a, b)

Note

When basal diameter and apical height do not fit this classification, the largest tumour diameter should be used for classification. In clinical practice, the tumour base may be estimated in optic disk diameters (dd) (average: 1dd = 1.5 mm). The height may be estimated in diopters (average: 3 diopter = 1.0 mm). Techniques such as ultrasonography are frequently used to provide more accurate measurements.

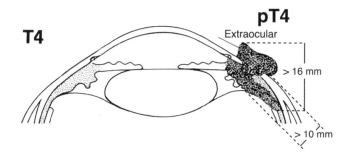

Fig. 474

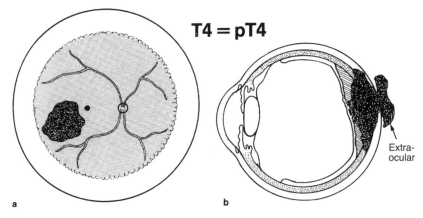

a   b

Fig. 475a, b

pT Pathological Classification

The pT categories correspond to the T categories.

Summary

Uvea Malignant Melanoma	
Iris Malignant Melanoma	
T1	Limited to iris
T1a	Iris ≤3 clock hours
T1b	Iris >3 clock hours
T1c	Iris with melanomalytic glaucoma
T2	Confluent with or into ciliary body/choroid
T2a	with melanomalytic glaucoma
T3	Scleral extension
T3a	with melanomalytic glaucoma
T4	Extraocular extension
Ciliary Body and Choroid Malignant Melanoma	
T1	≤10 mm basal, ≤2.5 mm height
T1a	without extraocular extension
T1b	with microscopic extraocular extension
T1c	with gross extraocular extension
T2	>10 to 16 mm basal, >2.5 to 10 mm height
T2a	without extraocular extension
T2b	with microscopic extraocular extension
T2c	with gross extraocular extension
T3	>16 mm basal and/or >10 mm height
T4	T3 with extraocular extension
All Sites	
N1	Regional

Retinoblastoma (ICD-O C69.2)

Rules for Classification

In bilateral cases, the eyes should be classified separately. The classification does not apply to complete spontaneous regression of the tumour. There should be histological confirmation of the disease in an enucleated eye.

T Clinical Classification

T—Primary Tumour

TX   Primary tumour cannot be assessed
T0   No evidence of primary tumour

T1   Tumour confined to the retina (No vitreous seeding or significant retinal detachment, or subretinal fluid over 5 mm from tumour base) (Fig. 476)

   T1a   Any eye in which the largest tumour is less than or equal to 3 mm in height *and* no tumour is located closer than 1 DD (1.5 mm) to the optic nerve or fovea (Fig. 477a, b)

   T1b   All other eyes in which the tumour(s) are confined to the retina regardless of location or size (up to half the volume of the eye).

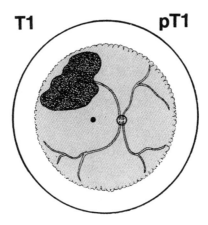

Fig. 476

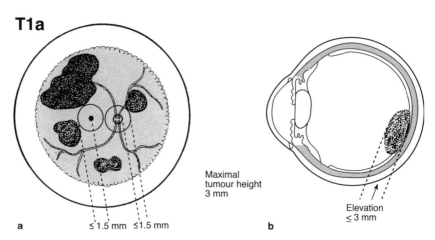

Fig. 477a, b

T2   Tumour with contiguous spread to adjacent tissues or spaces (vitreous or sub-
      retinal spaces)

    T2a   Minimal tumour spread to vitreous and/or subretinal space. Fine local
      or diffuse vitreous seeding and/or serous retinal detachment up to
      total detachment may be present, but no clumps, lumps, snowballs or
      avascular masses in the vitreous or subretinal space. Calcium flecks in
      the vitreous or subretinal space are allowed. The tumour may fill up
      to 2/3 the volume of the eye (Fig. 478).

    T2b   Massive tumour spread to vitreous and/or subretinal space. Vitreous
      seeding and/or subretinal implantation may consist of lumps, clumps,
      snowballs, or avascular tumour masses. Retinal detachment may be
      total. Tumour may fill up to 2/3 the volume of the eye (Fig. 479).

    T2c   Unsalvageable intraocular disease. Tumour fills more than 2/3 of the
      eye (Fig. 480) *or* there is no possibility of visual rehabilitation *or* one
      or more of the following are present:
      - Tumour associated glaucoma, either neovascular or angle closure
      - Anterior segment extension of tumour
      - Ciliary body extension of tumour
      - Hyphema (significant)
      - Massive vitreous hemorrhage
      - Tumour in contact with lens
      - Orbital cellulitis-like presentation (massive tumour necrosis)

T2a

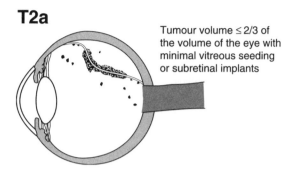

Tumour volume ≤ 2/3 of the volume of the eye with minimal vitreous seeding or subretinal implants

Fig. 478

T2b

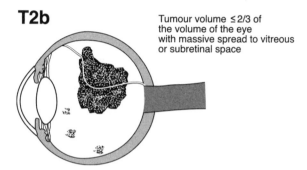

Tumour volume ≤ 2/3 of the volume of the eye with massive spread to vitreous or subretinal space

Fig. 479

T2c

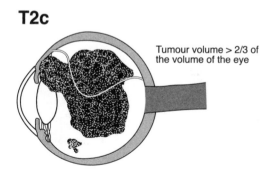

Tumour volume > 2/3 of the volume of the eye

Fig. 480

T3   Invasion of optic nerve and/or optic coats (Fig. 481a, b)
T4   Extraocular tumour (Fig. 482a, b)

Note
The suffix (m) may be added to the appropriate T categories to indicate multiple tumours, e.g., T2(m).

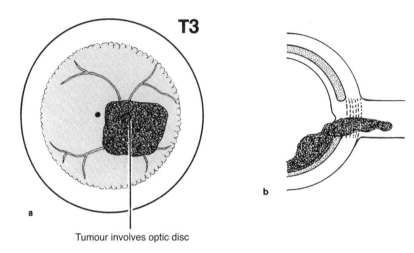

Tumour involves optic disc

Fig. 481a, b

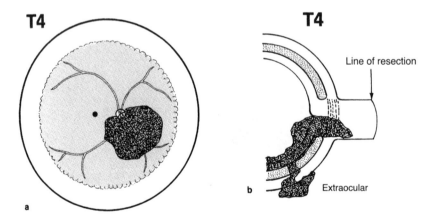

Fig. 482a, b

pT Pathological Classification

pT—Primary Tumour

pTX   Primary tumour cannot be assessed
pT0   No evidence of primary tumour

pT1   Tumour confined to the retina, vitreous, or subretinal space. No optic nerve invasion or choroidal invasion

pT2   Minimal invasion of the optic nerve and/or optic coats or focal invasion of choroid

    pT2a   Tumour invades optic nerve up to, but not through, the level of the lamina cribrosa

    pT2b   Tumour invades choroid focally

    pT2c   Tumour invades optic nerve up to, but not through, the level of lamina cribrosa *and* invades the choroid focally

pT3   Significant invasion of the optic nerve or optic coats or massive invasion of choroid

    pT3a   Tumour invades optic nerve through the level of lamina cribrosa but not the line of resection

    pT3b   Tumour massively invades to the choroid

    pT3c   Tumour invades the optic nerve through the level of lamina cribrosa but not to the line of resection *and* massively invades the choroid

pT4   Extraocular extension which includes any of the following:

- Invasion of optic nerve to the line of resection
- Invasion of orbit through the sclera
- Extension both anteriorly or posteriorly into the orbit
- Extension into the brain
- Extension into the subarachnoidal space of the optic nerve
- Extension to the apex of the orbit
- Extension to, but not through, the chiasm
- Extend into the brain beyond the chiasm

Editor's Note

Today enucleation of an eye for retinoblastoma is a rare event. Therefore, we have not included figures for the pT categories.

Summary

Retinoblastoma			
T1	Confined to retina	pT1	Retina, vitreous, or subretinal space
T1a	≤3 mm; not closer than 1 DD to optic nerve or fovea		
T1b	More than T1a		
T2	Intraocular tumour with contiguous spread to vitreous or subretinal space	pT2	Minimal invasion of optic nerve/coats
T2a	Minimal tumour spread to vitreous/subretinal space	pT2a	Optic nerve to, not through, lamina cribrosa
T2b	Massive tumour spread to vitreous/subretinal space	pT2b	Focal choroid invasion
T2c	Unsalvageable intraocular disease	pT2c	pT2a and b
T3	Optic nerve/optic coats invasion	pT3	Significant optic nerve/coats invasion
		pT3a	Through lamina cribrosa; not to resection line
		pT3b	Massive choroid invasion
		pT3c	pT3a and b
T4/pT4	Extraocular		
N1/pN1	Regional		
M1/pM1	Distant		
		pM1a	Bone marrow
		pM1b	Other sites

Sarcoma of Orbit (ICD-O C69.6)

Rules for Classification

The classification applies only to sarcomas of soft tissue and bone. There should be histological confirmation of the disease and division of cases by histological type.

T Clinical Classification

T—Primary Tumour

TX   Primary tumour cannot be assessed
T0   No evidence of primary tumour

T1   Tumour 15 mm or less in greatest dimension (Fig. 483)
T2   Tumour more than 15 mm in greatest dimension without invasion of globe or bony wall (Fig. 484)
T3   Tumour of any size with invasion of orbital tissues and/or bony walls (Fig. 485)
T4   Tumour invades globe or periorbital structures such as: eyelids, temporal fossa, nasal cavity/paranasal sinuses, and/or central nervous system (Fig. 486)

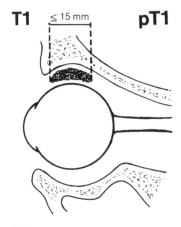

Fig. 483

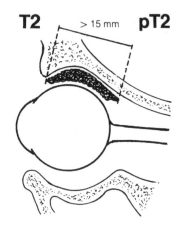

Fig. 484

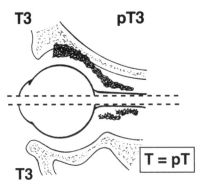

Fig. 485

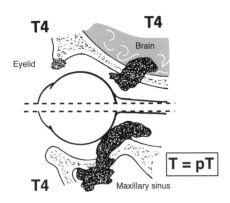

Fig. 486

pT Pathological Classification

The pT categories correspond to the T categories.

Summary

Sarcoma of Orbit	
T1	≤15 mm
T2	>15 mm
T3	Invades orbital tissues/bony walls
T4	Invades globe or periorbital structures
N1	Regional

Carcinoma of Lacrimal Gland

(ICD-O C69.5)

Rules for Classification

There should be histological confirmation of the disease and division of cases by histological type.

T Clinical Classification

T—Primary Tumour

TX	Primary tumour cannot be assessed
T0	No evidence of primary tumour

T1   Tumour 2.5 cm or less in greatest dimension, limited to the lacrimal gland (Fig. 487a, b)

T2   Tumour more than 2.5 cm, but not more than 5.0 cm, in greatest dimension, limited to the lacrimal gland (Fig. 488a, b)

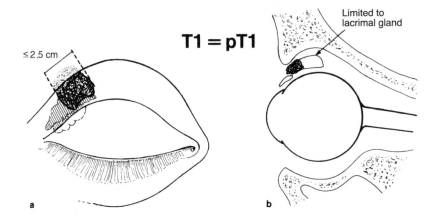

Fig. 487a, b

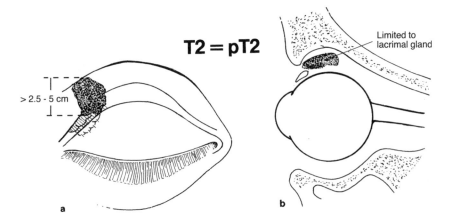

Fig. 488a, b

T3   Tumour invades periosteum
    T3a   Tumour not more than 5.0 cm, invades the periosteum of the lacrimal
            gland fossa (Fig. 489a, b)
    T3b   Tumour more than 5.0 cm in greatest dimension with periosteal invasion
            (Fig. 490a, b)

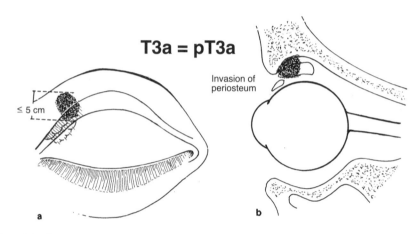

Fig. 489a, b

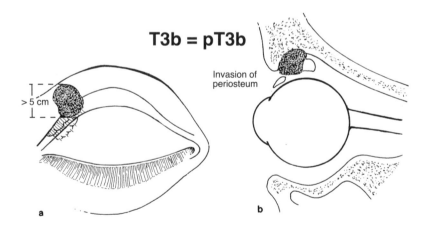

Fig. 490a, b

T4	Tumour invades the orbital soft tissues, optic nerve, or globe with or without bone invasion; tumour extends beyond the orbit to adjacent structures including brain (Figs. 491–492)

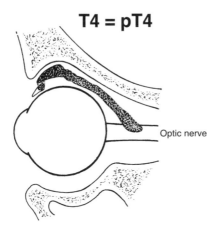

Optic nerve

Fig. 491

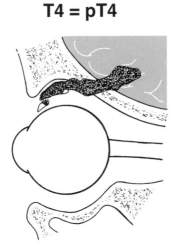

Fig. 492

pT Pathological Classification

The pT categories correspond to the T categories.

Summary

Lacrimal Gland Carcinoma	
T1	≤2.5 cm, limited to gland
T2	>2.5 to 5 cm, limited to gland
T3	Periosteum
T3a	Periosteum ≤5 cm
T3b	Periosteum >5 cm
T4	Orbit and beyond
N1	Regional

Hodgkin Lymphoma

Introductory Notes

At the present time it is not considered practical to propose a TNM classification for Hodgkin lymphoma.

Following the development of the Ann Arbor classification for Hodgkin disease in 1971, the significance of two important observations with major impact on staging has been appreciated. First, extralymphatic disease, if localized and related to adjacent lymph node disease, does not adversely affect the survival of patients. Secondly, laparotomy with splenectomy has been introduced as a method of obtaining more information on the extent of the disease within the abdomen[1].

A stage classification based on information from histopathological examination of the spleen and lymph nodes obtained at laparotomy cannot be compared with another without such exploration. Therefore, two systems of classification are presented, a clinical (cS) and a pathological (pS).

Editor's Note
[1] The same is valid for staging by laparoscopy.

Clinical Staging (cS)

Although recognized as incomplete, this is easily performed and should be reproducible from one centre to another. It is determined by history, clinical examination, imaging, blood analysis, and the initial biopsy report. Bone marrow biopsy must be taken from a clinically or radiologically non-involved area of bone.

Liver Involvement

Clinical evidence of liver involvement must include either enlargement of the liver and at least an abnormal serum alkaline phosphatase level and two different liver function test abnormalities, or an abnormal liver demonstrated by imaging and one abnormal liver function test.

Spleen Involvement

Clinical evidence of spleen involvement is accepted if there is palpable enlargement of the spleen confirmed by imaging.

TNM Atlas: Illustrated Guide to the TNM Classification of Malignant Tumours, Fifth Edition,
edited by Christian Wittekind, Frederick L. Greene, Robert Hutter, Martin Klimpfinger, and Leslie H. Sobin
Copyright © 2005 UICC

Lymphatic and Extralymphatic Disease

The lymphatic structures are as follows:

- Lymph nodes
- Waldeyer ring
- Spleen
- Appendix
- Thymus
- Peyer patches

The lymph nodes are grouped into regions and one or more (2, 3, etc.) may be involved. The spleen is designated S and extralymphatic organs or sites E.

Lung Involvement

Lung involvement limited to one lobe, or perihilar extension associated with ipsilateral lymphadenopathy, or unilateral pleural effusion with or without lung involvement but with hilar lymphadenopathy is considered as localized extralymphatic disease.

Liver Involvement

Liver involvement is always considered as diffuse extralymphatic disease.

Pathological Staging (pS)

This takes into account additional data and has a higher degree of precision. It should be applied whenever possible. A − (minus) or + (plus) sign should be added to the various symbols for the examined tissues, depending on the results of histopathological examination.

Histopathological Information

This is classified by symbols indicating the tissue sampled. The following notation is common to the distant metastases (or M1 categories) of all regions classified by the TNM system. However, in order to conform with the Ann Arbor classification, the initial letters used in that system are also given.

Pulmonary	PUL or L	Bone marrow	MAR or M
Osseous	OSS or O	Pleura	PLE or P
Hepatic	HEP or H	Peritoneum	PER
Brain	BRA	Adrenals	ADR
Lymph nodes	LYM or N	Skin	SKI or D
Others	OTH		

Clinical Stages (cS)

Stage I   Involvement of a single lymph node region (I) (Figs. 493–496), or localized involvement of a single extralymphatic organ or site (I$_E$) (Fig. 497)

cS: I   **pS: I**   **Fig. 493**

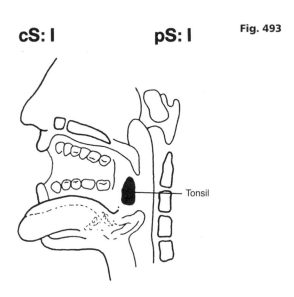

Tonsil

cS: I   **pS: I**   **Fig. 494**

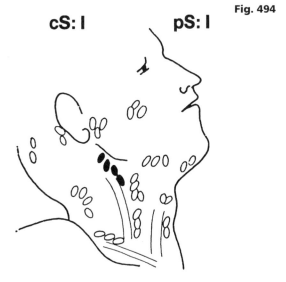

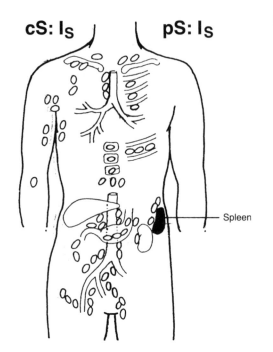

Fig. 495

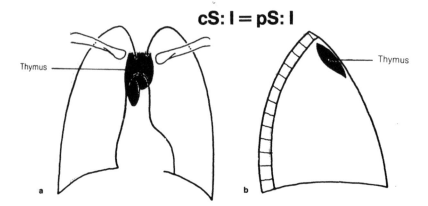

Fig. 496a, b

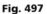
Fig. 497

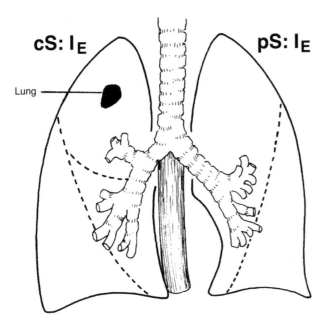

Stage II   Involvement of two or more lymph node regions on the same side of the diaphragm (II) (Fig. 498), or localized involvement of a single extralymphatic organ or site and its regional lymph node(s) with or without involvement of other lymph node regions on the same side of the diaphragm (II_E) (Fig. 499)

Note

The number of lymph node regions involved may be indicated by a subscript (e.g., II_3)

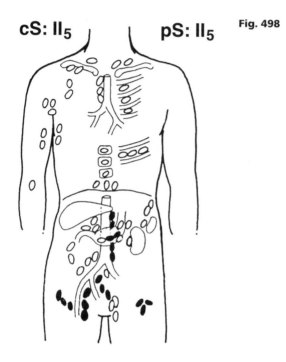

cS: II$_5$ pS: II$_5$ **Fig. 498**

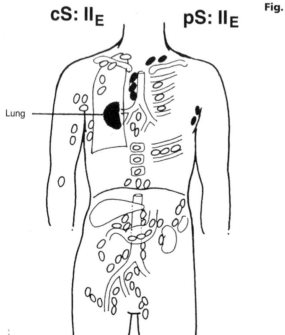

cS: II$_E$ pS: II$_E$ **Fig. 499**

Lung

Stage III   Involvement of lymph node regions on both sides of the diaphragm (III) (Fig. 500), which may also be accompanied by localized involvement of an associated extralymphatic organ or site (III$_E$) (Fig. 501a–c), or by involvement of the spleen (III$_S$), or both (III$_{E+S}$) (Fig. 502a, b)

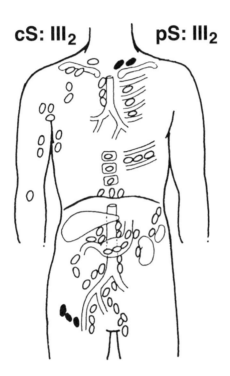

Fig. 500

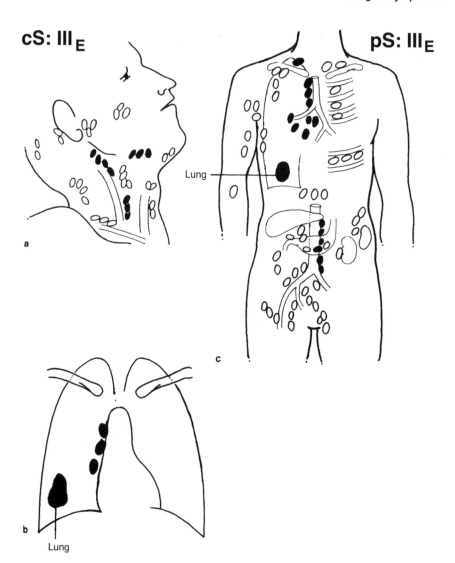

cS: III$_E$ pS: III$_E$

Lung

a

b   Lung

c

Fig. 501a-c

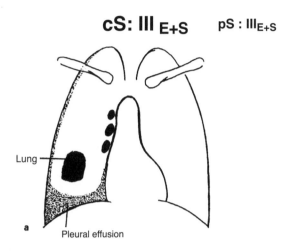

cS: III $_{E+S}$ pS : III$_{E+S}$

Lung

a   Pleural effusion

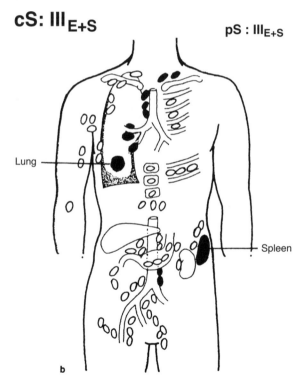

cS: III$_{E+S}$ pS : III$_{E+S}$

Lung

Spleen

b

Stage IV   Disseminated (multifocal) involvement of one or more
                  extralymphatic organs, with or without associated lymph node
                  involvement (Fig. 503–504a, b) or isolated extralymphatic organ
                  involvement with distant (non-regional) nodal involvement
                  (Fig. 505)

Note
The site of Stage IV disease is identified further by specifying sites according to the notations listed above.

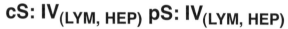

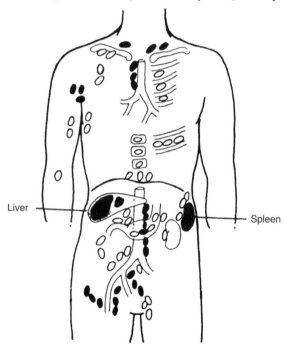

Fig. 503

$$\text{cS: IV}_{(LYM, PUL)}\text{pS: IV}_{(LYM, PUL)}$$

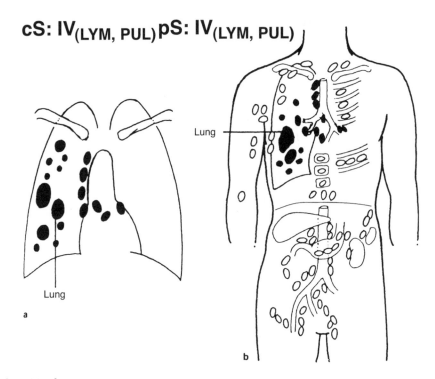

Fig. 504a, b

A and B Classification (Symptoms)

Each stage should be divided into A and B according to the absence or presence of defined general symptoms. These are:

1. Unexplained weight loss of more than 10% of the usual body weight in the 6 months prior to first attendance
2. Unexplained fever with temperature above 38 °C
3. Night sweats

Note
Pruritus alone does not qualify for B classification nor does a short, febrile illness associated with a known infection.

cS: IV$_{(LYM,HEP)}$ pS: IV$_{(LYM,HEP)}$

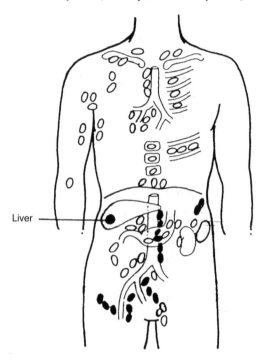

Liver

Fig. 505

Pathological Stages (pS)

The definitions of the four stages follow the same criteria as the clinical stages but with the additional information obtained following laparotomy or laparoscopy (see note p. 415). Splenectomy, liver biopsy, lymph node biopsy, and marrow biopsy are mandatory for the establishment of pathological stages. The results of these biopsies are recorded as indicated above (see p. 416).

Summary

Stage	Hodgkin Lymphoma	Substage
Stage I	Single node region	
	Localized single extralymphatic organ/site	I$_E$
Stage II	Two or more node regions, same side of diaphragm	
	Localized single extralymphatic organ/site with its regional nodes, $\pm$ other node regions same side of diaphragm	II$_E$
Stage III	Node regions both sides of diaphragm $\pm$ Localized single extralymphatic organ/site	III$_E$
	Spleen	III$_S$
	Both	III$_{E+S}$
Stage IV	Diffuse or multifocal involvement of extralymphatic organ(s) $\pm$ regional nodes; isolated extralymphatic organ and non-regional nodes	
All stages divided	Without weight loss/fever/sweats	A
	With weight loss/fever/sweats	B

Non-Hodgkin Lymphomas

As in Hodgkin disease, at the present time it is not considered practical to propose a TNM classification for non-Hodgkin lymphomas. Since no other convincing and tested staging system is available, the Ann Arbor classification is recommended with the same modification as for Hodgkin disease (see Figs. 493–505, pp. 416ff.)